Praise for *Tierra de mujeres*
Original Spanish edition

"Writer and veterinarian María Sánchez celebrates the women of her world, quiet workers of an ultrapatriarchal campaign. As indispensable as they are invisible. As omnipresent as they are silent. In this feminist and poetic manifesto, Sánchez draws on her own history to measure how much the earth is also a woman's affair."
  —*Le Monde*

"This book does not talk about the women who will fill the city streets. It speaks of a rural feminism…that remembers the strong and wise women who worked the land without raising their voices."
  —*Time Out*

"Narrated with agility, lucidity, forcefulness, and tenderness. There is knowledge, pride, vitality, and fantastic energy in this memoir about the women who, against the tide of history, didn't leave their family homes or their land, the ones who stayed with their men (or without them) in the rural area, the ones who resisted the exodus to the cities."
  —*El País*

"*Land of Women* is a beautiful tribute to the genealogy of women who came before, women with hands that molded the earth and who were part of the earth."

—*Heraldo de Aragón*

"María Sánchez asks us to consider the silent contribution of women in rural areas free from nostalgia, bucolic sentiments, and prejudice."

—*El Mundo*

"María Sánchez recovers the trace of the women in her life—in her learning, in the field, and in the home. As with the feminist movement, she turns our attention to that which was invisible to us until now."

—*Zenda*

"*Land of Women* launches a harangue against urban snobbery: no more stigmatizing the people of the countryside and ignoring their workers."

—*elDiario*

"Sánchez's ferocity echoes Elena Ferrante."

—*Asymptote*

"An expression of intimate and familiar memory endowed with great poetic strength."

—*ABC Sevilla*

"An essential [book] that focuses on the compelling need to expand feminist discourse so that it affects not only women in big cities but also those in rural areas. It deserves to be read by everyone. After all, there's still soil under the concrete."

—*La Vanguardia*

"Faced with a feminism that is highlighted through social media, María Sánchez knows that outside the cities, agriculture is an assumption without consideration. She gives feminist voice to the field."

—*El Cultural*

"*Land of Women* urges us to reconnect with the rural community, especially its women, and to tell our stories free of shame."

—*ABC Cultura*

"An epic book—political, pure, and sincere. There are few books as necessary as this."

—*El Confidencial*

"*Land of Women* is personal and unique—a book that cannot be defined under any one label. A book that is born from mourning. A book of trial and vindication. A book of intimate and collective memory."

—Anna María Iglesia

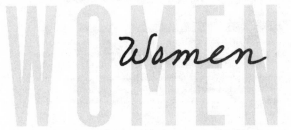

María
Sánchez

Translated by
CURTIS BAUER

Trinity University Press
SAN ANTONIO, TEXAS

Trinity University Press
San Antonio, Texas

978-1-59534-963-7 paperback
978-1-59534-964-4 ebook

Book design by BookMatters
Jacket design by Derek Thornton, Notch Design
Cover illustration: Joaquim Gomis, *Odette Gomis, Megève, France, 1939*.
Copyright © Hereus de Joaquim Gomis. Joan Miró Foundation, Barcelona.
Author photo by Cela Koto

Images on pages vi, 118, 134, and 150, copyright © Fernando Vílchez; page 54,
Grado Creativo Publicidad & Consulting; pages 16, 34, 74, 92, 108, 121, and 153,
author's personal collection; page 121, illustration from *Micrographia*, by Robert
Hooke (1665); page 153, from *Atlas of Human Anatomy and Surgery*, vol. 5, by
Jean-Baptiste Marc Bourgery, plate 72.

Trinity University Press strives to produce its books using methods and
materials in an environmentally sensitive manner. We favor working with
manufacturers that practice sustainable management of all natural resources,
produce paper using recycled stock, and manage forests with the best possible
practices for people, biodiversity, and sustainability. The press is a member
of the Green Press Initiative, a nonprofit program dedicated to supporting
publishers in their efforts to reduce their impacts on endangered forests,
climate change, and forest-dependent communities.

The paper used in this publication meets the minimum requirements of the
American National Standard for Information Sciences—Permanence of Paper
for Printed Library Materials, ANSI 39.48-1992.

CIP data on file at the Library of Congress

PRINTED IN CANADA

26   25   24   23   22   ≈   5   4   3   2   1

A mi familia

A aquellas y aquellos
que trabajaron y cuidaron la tierra
y nunca fueron reconocidos

Para ellos escribo

To my family

To those women and those men
who worked and cared for the land
and were never recognized

For them I write

CONTENTS

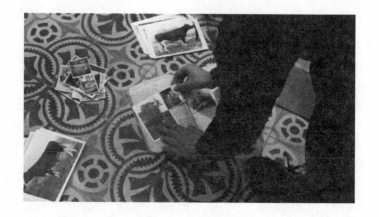

An Invisible Narrative

Could it be that inherited objects can be outlines of
our incomplete secrets?

—MARIA GABRIELA LLANSOL

Our grandparents' homes are full of portraits. They observe
us from behind the glass and it seems as if they might start
talking to us at any moment. Sometimes I think they're too
quiet. Other times, that they're scolding us with their gaze.
I like to stop and think about how those photographs were
made and why; who chose the scene, the frame, and that
ideal place for them to end up frozen in an instant, contemplating us from the wall. There's a certain care and ceremony that our most recent generations have left behind.
Today we can take a picture any time, anywhere we want,
but it has neither the value nor the ritualistic aura that it held
for our elders. There are no thought-out portraits, taken

calmly, with care. Those dedications that could be found on the back don't exist; there's no place for time to pass, for the color to yellow the hands and faces, the corners, the landscape. We, children of progress, no longer save photographs in albums or old cookie tins that were first sewing boxes and now are ending their days as a depository for faces and memories. Old framed photographs were a kind of sibling who lived among us, an intuition that averted its gaze as we passed, a need, sometimes real, for us to want to straighten them, dust them off, touch them, speak to them.

The way we look and our process of looking have also changed. It's no longer enough to raise our gaze to the walls to remember why one more element, technology, comes between the paper and our body. We rummage through computer applications, tools, systems, and social media so we can reminisce; we need some apparatus foreign to the ones we're thinking about in order to get closer to them. But truth is painful, and abrupt, if one stops to think about it. None of the people in the photographs hanging in the homes of our grandparents are alive now. There are only frames, empty frames.

It wasn't until the death of José Antonio, my paternal grandfather, the veterinarian, that I began to pause and dwell on the photographs that inhabited my two family homes. The questions began, the fear, the anxiety that I would continue my day-to-day life without knowing anything about the lives of those who came before me. It's interesting because José Antonio wasn't my first grandfather to die, but the second. José, my maternal grandfather, died when I was seven years old. Cancer took him too soon. He'd worked his whole life and the illness drowned him suddenly, like new puppies who can't swim and drown in a pool, without complaint or making a sound, without his realizing it. I was too young and I didn't notice it either. My only memory of him is of his bloody hands skinning hares in the yard behind his house. His shirt open, exposing his white undershirt, his pants held up with twine, his hands strong and tan, full of wrinkles, mixing with the animal's red entrails. I remember the heat clinging to our skin, some stray fly, a sweet kind of smell between life and death that overwhelmed the air itself, the clothesline, the flowerpots, and the stairs where he sat and turned into a figure that would appear again and again in my memory.

His death was a kind of process for me. Maybe because I'd hardly spent any time with him. He always seemed to be in the background. Now I wonder what would have happened if death had taken these men in a different order, if death had become a kind of solitary player that alters events and creates different paths through the lives of others. I can't help feeling a mix of anger and regret for not spending more time with him. It's something unconscious, that surges up without realizing it. Sometimes it seems like some kind of fiction.

Many years later, I woke up sweating, nervous, my heart pounding in my throat. It was extremely hot. I'd just had a dream, but I wouldn't remember it until hours later, when I was at work. Driving, coming back, not thinking about anything and only concentrating on the continuous line of the highway in front of me, suddenly, the images appeared. It was the first time I'd dreamed about my grandfather José. We were together, among his olive trees. In his hand, a little tree in a rusted, grime-covered can filled with dirt. On the ground, several freshly made holes, candidates to shelter and nourish the roots of a future olive tree, waiting, their anticipation punctuated by some stones. Hares ran between us, avoiding us as they left their burrows. We were just another element in the landscape, something that didn't interfere with or break the rhythm of the countryside. He spoke in the dream, but part of me knew it wasn't his voice. It's true that I let myself be carried away in the dream, only watching, my hands covered with dirt, holding the can with the little tree when he spoke. A mixture of grief and profound anger came over me while I was driving.

I'd forgotten his voice completely.

I often wonder if childhood is a mirage. I return to it so many times that I'm afraid I may have deformed or idealized it. For as long as I can remember, I've known that I wanted to grow up living like I did when I was a child. Becoming an adult by retracing my steps, returning to what surrounded me and made me feel so connected to the country. I am who I am because of my childhood. From an early age, I knew that I wanted to be a field veterinarian like my grandfather. I spent my childhood with him, among animals, in the garden. The rural environment was the essential substrate where my family, both maternal and paternal, has been rooted and prospering: our garden, root cellar, cork oaks, holm oaks, and olive trees; our siblings, animals, coworkers, and livelihood.

Those of us who write are often asked why we do what

we do. How does that first word emerge, the first poem, the first story. And we try, in vain, to explain something that has no boundaries, to make sense of it, to look for the root or origin of our obsession to express everything through words. I don't remember when I started to write, or why. In my head I imagine it as something automatic, routine, like someone looking for glasses, their hand fumbling across the bedside table after waking. It's something that has always been there. I could write about what makes me want to write. Those elements that suddenly become protagonists, hold the light and my attention, and that's it. Sometimes they appear and are with you for hours, days, even months, before they turn into words. I like to see them like a flash of light. Something that bursts in and illuminates, that changes the course of things.

My childhood is a flash of light: my grandparents' hands, the bindings and knives used for grafting, the motherless lambs, the goats coming to the shepherd's call, the olive trees and cork oaks, the cowbells, wool sweaters, my grandfather's veterinary books and manuals…Also what happens in my day-to-day life as a woman field veterinarian: the animals passing each other on the trails, the livestock producers—men and women—I work with, their words, their hands, the wicker baskets full of vegetables and eggs, the freshly boiled goat's milk, some *hijo*, or plant sprig or shoot plucked from one pot so it will grow in another, songs, stories, lullabies, little words you don't hear in cities and that here, thank goodness, roam freely and continue shifting through the hands of those who work and live on the land.

For the Portuguese writer Maria Gabriela Llansol, her garden at Herbais—her house in exile where she spent so many hours caring for the plants as she read, or just sitting, thinking—was her invisible narrative, the initial flash that later allowed the word to rise up so she could begin to write, as if that light springing from what obsesses us and excites us, in a certain way, moved into the hand that ends up tipping the word onto the page.

A question that haunts me is what would happen if this invisible narrative that is such a part of my life weren't this one. Would I write? Would I have a different one? This, so to speak, is my invisible narrative, and here I take shelter, and here, and like this, I try to build a home, still fragile, timid, sometimes body and sometimes spirit, where furrows, branches, animals and seeds, where the word, beating, trembling, seeks to remove shadow and dust from the rural environment and all the people who live there.

Another flash, one of the most recurring ones, is the trip we took and continue to take by car to our hometown, our pueblo. When I was little, my cheek always pressed to the glass, whether it was hot or cold, looking sideways, squinting and straining to see, sharpening my ear as well, as if I could cross through the window, counting live oaks between the holm oaks, bushes, and cork oaks, seeing the little animals crossing beyond the fingers and the attentive voices of my parents, the steps of some hesitant, always doubting deer on the side of the road, the rockroses spreading along the shoulder, scratching the car, as if they were reaching out to us. Counting was a way to make time pass more quickly, a way of wanting to know, calling to those animals that appeared in front of us. Substitute them for the minutes; turn them into the minute hand that never stops and was a complete stranger that emerged in our childhood. Maybe that's where I find a sort of calm, tranquility, unreal serenity, that little voice that tells me that everything is okay and that everything will be okay when I learn the name of something I don't know. I think it was George Steiner who wrote that "what isn't named doesn't exist." But who will continue to name those who cease to exist? Will they still be around despite the fact that they no longer exist and have ceased to be named? And who will name for the first time what isn't named? What sets off the first voice and the first name?

When my paternal grandmother Teresa's senile dementia appeared, I discovered that I knew nothing about her. Absolutely nothing. I tried to follow her trail, to question, to investigate. But I was also late. My grandmother had an eighty-some-year-old body and a spoiled brain that made her think she was still in her twenties. I wasn't her granddaughter; I was just another friend from the town. A companion to confide in and laugh with. My grandmother had turned into a kind of sassy young woman who laughed and talked to me about where she'd hide the letters boys had written her so her mother wouldn't find them. In a low voice she laid out plans for pranks; she told me where her mother hid her coin purse so that afternoon we could go to the plaza for ice cream. She talked about the beach, about a house with a giant piano. My grandfather, my father, and the rest of my uncles didn't exist, they didn't have any place in her photograph. Another empty frame.

She died, and with her death she left me with another obsession. That of rummaging through the trunks and dressers in my grandparents' houses in search of photographs. Not the ones that hang on the walls, the well-known ones, not those. I was obsessed with the ones that remained in the cookie tins, alone, piled up, stacked on top of each other, away from the light that destroys them, without voices to accompany them and look at them, without dressers and desks to rest upon. They became the ones I questioned. In them I was looking for everything I had allowed to pass by without realizing, like someone who starts driving a car down a path and doesn't realize that it's the trees that are leaving, not us. And they leave without saying a word, not bothering to look back, without a word remaining, swaying on the path. They go away and leave us; they don't wait for us to realize time is passing by. That minute hand keeps moving, despite the animals on the shoulders of the highway, the little birds crisscrossing each other, those waiting for us to point at them with our finger, to ask about them, to name them.

With the death of my three grandparents the rooms became empty. The chairs ridiculous, the pantries useless, the pots silenced in the shadows, the vestibules closed, pointless. The frames empty, once again. And not only in these houses, but in so many, and so many that are closed when the last of the living there are forced to leave and they cover their furniture with sheets, like someone who closes the eyes of the one who dies, that act that's only done once, that is born and dies in an instant, knowing, like a wound is born, like a certainty is formed, that no one will ever come back to uncover them.

This is my invisible narrative. My home, in flames, that never waits for the last brick or for the word to be ready to be inhabited. Is this what writing is? Something you never expect? That comes up suddenly and imposes itself?

It's reasonable to acknowledge the similarity and change of rhythm between writing, life in rural areas, and the life that is imposed upon us at this moment. Other tones, other songs, other rhythms. In literature just like in the country, I believe, there shouldn't be immediacy. Two worlds that, at first, seem so far apart, share so much. The flashes, the seeds, the care, the calm, the patience while you watch all the multitudes that are born grow, care for them, and they expand and continue to do so regardless. Beautiful or cruel, they are the result of a caring hand and have the same goal: survival.

My grandparents had to disappear from my life for me to realize it. A little late, because children and grandchildren are always late for things, for life itself. As much as our fathers and mothers tell us, prepare the way for us, give us clues to see the bird we sense on the branch, but do not see. And we can't see it because we are slow to learn to look, to settle our gaze and know how to touch along the edges, to realize that behind the little frames that hang in the houses of our grandmothers and mothers there's an uncomfortable beauty, an ache, a history, a latent genealogy waiting for us to rescue it and make it our own. A genealogy where we belong and can recognize ourselves.

The essay that grows from here, like the coiled pods of wild clover clinging to the rumps of the transhumant sheep in order to germinate a thousand miles from the place where they were born, is simply that, an arrival, one that I hope isn't too late, to what makes up my invisible narrative; an arrival to those women who were not named and existed, to those women who are still there in the shadows, with a voice, though one we don't hear because there is no possible space or *altavoz*—no sound system for them to make themselves heard. This essay is a hand, in the end, determined to reach out and transplant, to take care of, before the little frames in our homes become completely orphaned, silent, empty, without anyone to look at them.

PART
ONE

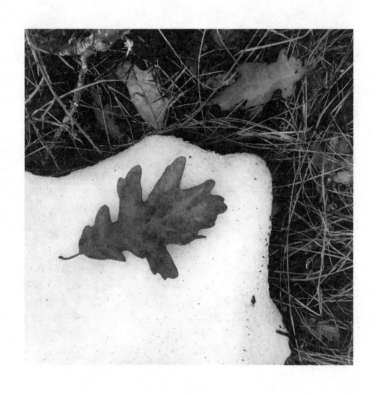

CHAPTER 1

A Genealogy of the Countryside

I am the sister of an only child.

—AGUSTINA BESSA-LUÍS

I come from a land where snow is unfamiliar. We are used to the electricity going out, the television signal disappearing and the screen reflecting only what the candlelight illuminates. An unusable object that becomes the mirror of those of us who are sitting at the table, playing with the butterfly candles, those butterflies that never fly, only float, which are kept in a wrinkled cardboard box protected by a drawing of a saint, lulled by the smell and heat across our knees under the table skirt, by the sound of the poker in the *brasero de picón*, the coal-warming pan. Life goes on, our elbows resting on the tabletop while the lights in the house come back on.

My maternal grandmother, Carmen, the only grandmother I have left, is scared to death of storms. She doesn't
like it when the rest of us are away from the house while it's
raining and there are thunderstorms. I don't know who in
my family told me that when she was young and it would
begin to storm, she would place a jar of salt with scissors
stuck inside it under the bed so that nothing would happen
to the house or any of its inhabitants. I've never known why.
I've never asked her. As if that ritual were perfectly normal, a rite to celebrate at home, something deeply rooted,
familiar.

We are attracted by what we don't understand. When it
snows in my town, we observe it in a unique way. We go out
in the street, we throw snowballs at each other, we go up to
the helicopter pad and we throw ourselves down the slope
using plastic bags for sleds; we get in the car and we go to
the fields, to see how the animals are managing in this new
element, to check the finger depth of the quilt that covers
the ground.

In my job, when I drive north and suddenly find myself surrounded by snow, I can't stop looking at it. It becomes a

magnet. Sometimes I feel the need to touch it. But it's hard to stop if you're driving on the highway. You're only allowed to do so at some clearly marked area built specifically for stopping: it's not actually the countryside, but something artificial, a rest area where the landscape ceases to be what it looked like from inside the windshield. The lanes that lead out to the pastures and farmland, to places where cows graze and their shadows are confused with the trees when night falls, are never signposted. Then a feeling of disappointment appears because what you long for has another form; it doesn't exist. Suddenly, the snow in that rest area seems trivial, out of place, meaningless. Your breathing adapts to the speed of the cars on the road. The moisture soaks your feet, reminding you that you are a stranger in an equally strange place. You know there is a herd because of their bells, a town because of the chimney smoke, a bird by the sound of a sudden flutter. You approach the trees looking for a small nest among the branches, but you know you won't find anything. You look at the ground and there are no tracks other than your own footprints. What you'd seen when you were driving has been left behind, in the rearview mirror, turned into something unattainable. You are out of place. You are in the country, but at the same time the country doesn't exist. There are no animals or houses, no nests or tracks. The trees were planted in the same way that the picnic tables and trash containers were planted. There is no interrelationship between them and the environment that surrounds them.

> A rest area. Just one more illusion that shatters as we approach it from the car. A mirage. Nowhere.

I don't put jars of salt under the bed when a storm comes up, but I can't help imagining those who live outside squaring off against it. I reside in what happens in the rearview mirror when I'm traveling. I become a mere spectator. I imagine those who are outside, fleeing the trees, giving in to the snow or rain, running, back home. I also ask myself about the animals; I speculate about how the change of weather affects them. I think a lot about nests. Will the young notice the first drops of rain? Will they be aware of the branches rocking in the air? Will they recognize the snow, the rain, the wind? Will they have that same irremediable attraction that I feel whenever it starts to snow?

I had to write and publish a book, *Field Notebook*, so that my family's stories could begin to walk by themselves through the house without fear or shame. And I didn't do it consciously—I mean, at home things occurred and happened without my paying attention to them or thinking about them. My parents and my grandparents maybe thought that what they had to tell me wasn't good enough or that interesting. And now I'm a little embarrassed to realize that as children we didn't dare to ask. I saw, I listened, I let things happen, I imitated. But it was hard for me to ask about those close to me, about what happened in the fields, about the names of trees and animals, about seeds, about jars and recipes. Since I didn't know how my schoolmates lived in their homes, I thought their lives would be just as full of the same elements as mine. I was wrong. Not everyone has a hometown. Not everyone can return to a piece of land and hike up their skirts to collect food from the garden. Call the flock which comes running to the sound of that voice. And since I didn't share that substratum of life with them, I isolated myself. And since I didn't ask or want to know, I'd run to my books and find the answers there, unconscious, naive, not knowing that the answers were much closer than I thought.

Always, there are always tracks.

And that's why, when I sense the snow in the distance or the flakes begin to fall when I'm heading north, I always think of the same scene that I read about in the book *Peasant's Prayer* by Eliseo Bayo that emerged from the interviews he did in the 1960s and '70s with the people who worked and lived in this nation's rural areas.

The image from Eliseo's book that always comes back to me when the snow blows in belongs to a custom common among the transhumant shepherds of the north. When it snowed or rained, they changed the way they stepped on the ground. One would lead the way, while the rest adopted the habit of stepping in the footprints of the first one in order to avoid getting their feet wet. It was a matter of survival. So, footprint after footprint, they continued, until it was time to eat. Then, the body, out in the open, would look for shelter among the warm breath of the flock, in those small circles in the shapes of animals that, at nightfall, dapple the ground. The land, warm and finite, gave a few hours' respite to the travelers before they set off again.

Maybe the root cause is there: although the snow is so strange to me, I can't help but make it mine. And I glance back and look again, I walk on my tiptoes over the tracks, I look at my father and my grandfather, I recognize myself as a girl, attentive and aware of what they were doing, and I feel like that transhumant shepherd who places his feet very carefully in the footprints that the one before has so firmly marked.

Because, by habit, we usually learn from the one who precedes us, from the one who got his feet wet first. And as in so many families and stories that come to pass in this country, in a certain way, the ones who have been opening the way for us, stepping the water out of the track and clearing the brambles from the path so that the flock can continue on, have been men. Those men. The first ones. Those who were seen. The ones who could be pointed out. Recognized. Appreciated. Men we want to be like.

I acknowledge this:

I am a woman who is a third generation: my grandfather was a veterinarian, my father is a veterinarian, and so am I. I am the first granddaughter, the first daughter, the first niece. But also *la primera veterinaria*, the first woman veterinarian. I come from a family that has always been linked to the land and to animals, to extensive livestock production. My childhood is full of cork oaks, holm oaks and olive trees, a few vegetable gardens, root cellars and a lot of animals. As a child, I always looked up to them. The men were the voice and the arm of the house. In fact, I wanted to be one of them. As a little girl and until I was well into my teens, I hated dresses, the hair my mother insisted I wear long and comb, and the dolls I was supposed to play with. I wanted to be strong, I ran fearlessly behind the herd, and I fell again and again when I bravely steered around the tracks, too wide for my bike, which remained in the lanes a while after the tractors passed. I was always the first one to appear when my grandfather or my father needed help. I wanted to be like them. To show them that I was as strong and as ready as they were. Because if there is something that is clear to us from a young age it is this. Men of blood and earth never cry, they are not afraid, they are never wrong. They always know what needs to be done. Always.

At that age, the women in my home were like ghosts who roamed the house, appearing and disappearing. They were invisible. Sisters of an only child, as the Portuguese writer Agustina Bessa-Luís once said about her childhood. Sisters of strong men. Invisible women in the shadow of a brother. In the shadow and at the service of a brother, a father, a husband, of their own sons. And this couldn't be more accurate and, at the same time, more painful. Because this is the story of our country and of so many others: women who remained in the shadows and without a voice, orbiting around the star of the house, who kept quiet and gave in; loyal, patient, good mothers, cleaning gravesites, sidewalks, and facades, saturating their hands with whitewash and lye every year; knowers of remedies, ceremonies, and lullabies; witches, teachers, sisters, speaking softly among themselves, becoming shelter and nourishment; turning into, over the years, another unnoticed room, into an artery inherent to the house.

But who are the ones telling the stories of women? Who worries about rescuing our grandmothers and mothers from that world they were confined to, from that quiet room, in miniature, reducing them to mere companions, exemplary wives and good mothers? Why have we normalized a narrative of our history where they are not participants? Who has seized their spaces and voice? Who really writes about them? Why aren't these women the ones who write about our rural community?

Many things have had to happen and a lot of time has had to pass so I could know the stories of the women in my family, to be able to delve into them, recognize myself there and feel proud. To be unashamed to ask questions and get to know them, and also know myself, after all. The houses have had to remain empty, absurd with their little picture frames, with their subjects always looking at me. Many of the women in my family have had to go away and never come back. Sometimes without looking back, without leaving even the faintest trace on the ground for us to follow in their footsteps. Maybe as daughters we have woken up a bit late, but at last we are questioning and making demands; we are using our voices to take control. Now that I look back and think about it, I can't help noticing a feeling like a wall clock pendulum swinging between rage and guilt. Why didn't women occupy a prominent place among my mentors? Why weren't they ever the example I wanted to follow? Why, as a child, didn't I want to be like them?

It seems strange, now that we are fortunate to live in a feminist society, to ask such obvious questions. But looking back at our homes we find similar stories. Everything that entered the house—the important, the joyous, and the great achievements, the good news—always came from the same voice. They told us that the man was the only one who worked, that he was the one who deserved to rest when he got home. We silenced and moved to the shadows those who did the housework, those who rolled up their sleeves and skirts in our towns, those who helped with the farrowing, those who worked in the garden, took care of the chickens, picked olives; we put them in the shadows. They were removed from the light so that the center of attention and the foundations of the house always illuminated the man, so the rest of us wouldn't look away, or lose our focus. We understood, as a matter of course, that our mothers and grandmothers would take care of everything and could do everything: the house, the caregiving, the children, the fields, the animals. We took away their stories and thought nothing of it. We let the men be the ones to speak, those who continued to lead the way for the rest of us. These women, our grandmothers, our mothers, our aunts, we saw them as something both strange and familiar, something close but belonging to another galaxy, with another sense of time and another demeanor. They talked to us and told us things, but we didn't understand them, because we simply didn't listen to them. The standards that we'd been given to that point were established almost entirely by the male gender.

How do you write about what you don't value? How do you remove from the shadow what is placed there and left there as if it were something normal? How do you rewrite women? How do you give them back the voice and the words they've always had but which have not been heard or even considered? How can we include them in our stories if in our language and our narratives they've never held a protagonist's role?

Not everything is reduced to the domestic sphere. This isolation of women is a disease that has managed to spread through all strata. I feel like someone who discovers rooms in an abandoned house and goes in, room by room lifting the sheets that cover the furniture, and looks for a reflection in the windows and mirrors. No. It's not just the house I grew up in. The infection reached every layer of my life: school, university, my job.

The books surrounding me as I grew up, all those notes and reference manuals I spent so many hours with in the library, animal and bird guides, all those novels, stories, and poems, everything, practically in their entirety, written by the same sex. All those I admired and followed: scientists, ecologists, thinkers, veterinarians, shepherds, farmers, day laborers, livestock producers, conservationists, educators, all of them, everyone, absolutely all of them, men.

My grandfather. My father. My uncles. Those who worked in the fields and those I was close to so I could be like them. The hours glued to the television watching the documentaries of Félix Rodríguez de la Fuente. So many passages by Miguel Delibes. The poems of Federico García Lorca. Wanting to write like Julio Llamazares when I first read *Yellow Rain*. The animals that never stopped howling in the poems by Ted Hughes. The birds that lived with a quote from Shakespeare in Peterson's guide. Like the birds that John Audubon killed to then be able to more easily paint them. Castejón, the humanist and veterinarian from Córdoba. Also the one who was president of the republic in exile, and who became the first veterinarian to recognize and value the livestock native to our land: Gordón Ordás. That endearing saga full of creatures great and small by the Englishman James Herriot. My grandfather's old veterinary books and manuals in French, always written by men. Like the pictures of cows he brought back from his trips to Canada. There were always smiling men who posed with their animals in these photographs: the protagonists, owners, caretakers.

Where were the women?

I know that what I just outlined may seem too obvious. Ten years ago, maybe even less, it wasn't like that. Fortunately, I belong to a brilliant generation that has a crucial task: to rescue all those women who have been pushed aside over the years, left alone, without remorse, without a voice, like those pieces of furniture in some empty houses together with the moths, covered by a useless sheet that offers no protection. It only makes them invisible. It only extinguishes their voice. Thanks to this collective awakening, thanks to feminism, a tireless and necessary search emerges. At last, we are getting to know women scientists, writers, activists, thinkers, ecologists, conservationists…women who moved and stood out in a world of men but who, because they were women, went completely unnoticed.

Fortunately, today the roles have changed: the stories of women are coming to light and becoming reference points, offering role models to follow and lives that matter for girls today and for those to come. When we begin to be aware of how important it is to recognize ourselves in someone, a new feeling emerges: to feel like the sister of someone who knows the way. We can turn her into a key element in our history, into part of the apparatus that will allow us to grow day by day. A path to extend and create, at last, our own narrative.

We want women in all areas and spaces.

They should be the ones who narrate, teach, and build. They should be the ones who can move forward without feeling afraid or ashamed. It's something that we now think is completely normal in our daily lives. We get angry if we notice that there are no women wherever we are in any kind of event. We speak out, we write, we take to the streets, we celebrate.

And I, a woman who comes from a rural community and who works in it, today I feel like that swinging pendulum on the wall clock. Like a rope that falls away but is at the same time attached. Like that bucket we lower into the well without knowing what it will bring up to us when we raise it to the light.

Because I'm trying to build a home. A home to shelter all those *destellos*, those flashes that have brought me here. Some foundations and some walls that give sanctuary to words, to lullabies, to animals. So I can feel accompanied, not by ghosts, not by shadows. So I feel safe to talk about where I come from and where I live. But whenever I start to lay the next brick, the same thing happens: the house I was building was only full of men.

My invisible narrative. The women in my house. Like the shadowy area, that part of the mountainside the sun hardly reaches. Those slopes that, due to their orography, remain steadfast to the shade.

Strong species also grow in the shade. Trees and plants that need more water. Animals that search it out for shelter and for nourishment. Like men in summer who sit in it to rest between work and chores. The shadow. The absence of light. That we can't see them, or rather, that we don't know how to see them, doesn't mean that they aren't there.

> Is it possible that besides our name, we need light to exist?

I go back to that home project and look around. I search in my books, on my shelves, in newspaper clippings. I read what others wrote about rural communities before. What others write about rural communities now. And I stumble. I stumble again and again over that literature that calls us farmers, which always associates us with the empty word, which describes us out of that patronizing attitude and from the big cities, which visit us for their funny news stories, which insist on writing about the rural community as if they were gravediggers appropriating the voice of those whose hands are smudged with dirt and inhabit the countryside and mountains. Nor do they, what a surprise, mention *ellas*, the women.

Our rural community needs other hands to write about it, hands that do not claim to rescue it or situate it. Hands that know about the sunny spots and the shade, about light and shadow. About what is heard and what is intuited. About what trembles and what is not named.

A narrative that rests in the footprints. In the footprints of all those women who wore out their espadrilles walking and working, in the shadow, without making noise, and who remain alone, waiting for someone to recognize them and begin to name them into existence.

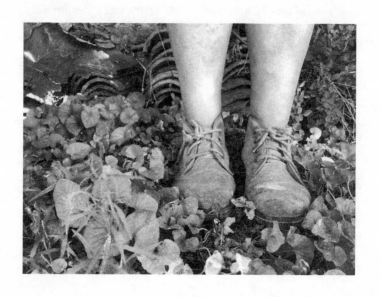

CHAPTER 2

A Feminism of Sisters and Land

The woman said: Lord,
since the beginning of time
you have placed me at the feet of the living
and at the bedside of the dead.

—NATHAN ALTERMAN

Indifference does not exist in small towns. Everyone knows each other here. Everyone knows about the good and the bad. Everyone has a part in the stories that are told and those that stay inside the home. You can't be invisible in a small town; you can't stop existing. Lives and death follow each other in a totally different way than they do in the city. They become a ceremony that also belongs to the town; the community is part of them—it gets involved, in a kind of celebration. The inhabitants speak openly about those who are born and those who die, recounting all kinds of details, making you a part of what happens on their streets. They talk about death like they talk about rain and cold, like someone who hopes for good weather. In towns, unlike cities, death is not hidden. Death dirties, reaches the bells and the doors, leaves its smell and its touch in the rooms. It's just another passer-by who walks the streets, who recognizes knocks at all the neighbors' doors. It's just one more dinner guest who sits at the table, who doesn't eat or drop its napkin when it sits down, who never asks for seconds but also never gets up, who is always there, silent, attentive, present.

Weeks before Día de Todos Los Santos, All Saints' Day, the women roll up their sleeves and prepare to tidy up the places where their loved ones, those who are no longer around, live. They go to the cemetery loaded down with ladders and buckets full of rags and bottles of cleaning products. They clean the graves, polish the tombstones, paint the walls of their little plots, change the vases, bring new flowers for their dead. They talk, talk a lot with the dead as they do these little chores in the cemeteries. Since I was a little girl, I always found it odd to hear the women in my town, to sense in them, especially my mother, my grandmother, and my aunts, a kind of worry that they hadn't gone to the section of the family burial plot they were in charge of before November 1 to make sure it was clean. Their family, those who are no longer here but are still among us, those who look at us from the photographs, from some frame tilted under the weight of their absence, those who still have a name but no body or voice, those we continue to name, missing, imagining them in present situations and raising possibilities that would never take place if they were here. As if those, our loved ones, were reviewing this work and noticed their absence.

And those buried in the cemeteries, what do they know? Do they know that there are sister gravesites of their own, those that no one tends to and no one talks to, that are left alone and give way to soft green grass that spreads over them like a fine blanket? Will they notice the hands of their family protected by plastic gloves, the smell of bleach and the rattle of the ladders and the replacement of the flowers? Will they and the always-present cypress trees notice the last ones to arrive? Will the cleaning by those hands and those new lilies look anything like relief?

What those who leave and those who come to the towns do and don't do is no secret; everything is known. Everything can become an open secret. Everyone knows about everyone else, for better or for worse. And any kind of exposure, like coming into the open or raising one's voice, is also a way of standing out.

I remember the first time I heard the popular expression "Small town, big hell." It was a shock, a contradiction with myself. In part, because something about it makes sense. When the community is small, there are links between everyone, innate ties that unite and tighten among its inhabitants. And like everything that transpires and pulses, it has its good things and others that aren't so good. But something in me also rebuked this popular saying, which I thought was unfair. Could it be that we are experts in bringing to light only the bad? In pointing out what should matter less? Does everything that happens in a town fit into those four words?

Some time later, this contradiction is still with me. For everything it entails, for the times we are living in and that are ultimately here to stay. March 8, 2018, clearly marked a before and after for women, for the country, even reaching all the cities across the territory. The streets and the plazas turned into a celebration, a party. Women of all generations took to the streets to raise their voices, to be seen like never before. I was also part of that much-needed, light-filled purple tide. We shook hands, voices became one, women all together; even if we didn't know each other, we recognized each other, we supported each other. We were sisters.

The media outlets were filled with feminist proclamations and manifestos. Hair-raising videos and photos of the demonstrations were shared. Tears were shed; it was impossible not to be moved by what we experienced in this country on March 8. Days before, many women from different sectors got organized. They organized the strike, formed groups, gave instructions. They supported each other. Every time I went online I found a new manifesto: women journalists, writers, editors, doctors, lawyers, nurses. It was clear to all these women in all these different professions that they had to go on strike. They joined forces, they united, they embraced each other. On March 8 women made the streets tremble. Many, although they couldn't join the strike and demonstrations, hung their aprons outside their windows. A crowd walking confidently together became a single voice.

That day I also felt a little out of place and the contradiction returned. I became a little orphaned from other sisters. I have to admit that I was angry when I saw that there were so few women who joined the strike and took to the streets in rural towns. Where were the women?

In my day-to-day life as a field veterinarian, I'm surrounded by wonderful women; I work with them and they have a lot to say and teach me. Women who care for our rural community and who make our food and the potential of our territory possible. Women who, with their own hands, open the way, mark a new path to food sovereignty. Country women, livestock producers, day laborers, farmers, artisans, shepherds, all women. The same women who leave the doors of their houses open so their neighbors can come in whenever they want, who share what they gather in their garden or any food that comes into their home, all those women who live in our towns. Women I barely saw in the photographs and videos of the demonstrations. Women who didn't appear in any manifesto. I felt sorrow, a mixture of sadness and rage. I couldn't understand. Where was the gap? Why were some streets so crowded and other plazas so empty?

I work in two worlds, the rural and the cultural, which I try to learn how to balance so that they get along with each other, even if they have their conflicts, even if these two worlds take time away from each other, even if they often contradict each other. The writer part of me was thrilled by all the feminist manifestos and the whole movement and support from the cultural world for the strike on March 8. But what about my other side? Where did I have to look to find that same strength and shelter?

Once again the tracks of those who have gone before us and the mirrors they are reflected in are important. Footsteps, the times, the rhythms, the distances. Like this excerpt from the trilogy *Into Their Labours* by John Berger:

> For country people, distance is a relative notion that depends on their method of cultivating the earth. If they grow melons between the cherry trees, five hundred meters is a considerable distance. If they graze cattle in a mountain pasture, five kilometers isn't so far.

Only when you stop and look around do you really learn how to see differently. To recognize what is there and what isn't seen but also exists. And that it has other forms and follows a different time frame. On March 8, on the street and surrounded by women who felt like a real family, I noticed that a large part of my roots and my companions were missing. *Ellas* weren't there—the women. They were absent. The women from our rural areas. Their absence was painful. It unsettled me, made me angry, sad. Because it is when we learn to recognize ourselves in someone else that we can also feel like we exist for ourselves. I was hurt by that lack of representation of women from our towns, from the rural community. An absence of a fair and more than necessary recognition for all of them.

But we forget that the country has another concept of time, other rhythms. And that urban feminism cannot demand a specific form and speed from rural feminism. In the city you can walk down the street and no one recognizes you. Being seen, raising your voice, speaking out doesn't mean anything most of the time. Today I think about those women who went out to the plazas in their towns and I was sad that there were so few. How wrong I was. I had no right to get angry with them, to reproach them for anything. The act of demonstrating and going on strike in a small town takes on more relevance and involves much more than in a city. Because they all know each other. Everyone talks the next day. Everybody points. And those few women who marched out in force in their towns meant and mean a great deal. Distances, seeds, time. What they germinated last March 8, however small it was, is growing and begining to come to the surface. And it's bursting forth with strength and voice. And it's already here, creating a beautiful network for the women of the land.

Possibly many on this side felt like I did that day. With that mixture of happiness and helplessness. The part of me that works with the rural community, my veterinarian self, stood completely alone in the face of the conflict. Because we aren't aware of how important it is to feel supported, to be part of a group, to feel the warmth of recognition. To look around you and see yourself in the face of another woman who is shaking your hand and smiling at you. Who tells you, without speaking, that she is there, with you. That's why all those women who marched out to the plazas in their towns were a small victory. Even if they only went out and allowed themselves to be seen. Some may have gone on strike, but I know that many didn't even consider it. Because the decision to stop, to move ahead with the strike, isn't only an individual matter, but it forms part of a balance, where, I insist, group, recognition, and identity are absolutely essential.

Rural women start from a different place than urban women. The rural community in this country continues to be that stranger we never end up getting close to. We continue to write about our rural environment from the big cities, falling into some idealization, in that flat and bucolic postcard that never seems to break apart. The country I move and work in has very little to do with the one portrayed with sentimentality, even with a kind of nostalgia in the media. It's wonderful to see that rural areas are *in fashion*, but seeing a wave of summer and weekend newspaper columnists without any connection to or serious concern for our rural community creates a feeling of powerlessness. Because here we start from the bottom. The inhabitants of the towns are second-class citizens. I don't shudder when I write that. From the perspective of the cities the fact that people in our towns don't have the same access to basic services seems normal. Health, education, culture, infrasctructure. Those who, in spite of everything, want to stay, we have left to fend for themselves. And the last thing these rural men and women need is a *rural* literature to rescue them. Because they don't need to be saved. They need schools, good roads, and health centers. They need the administration to help them and support them, not to mistreat them. They need initiatives to choose from, so they aren't forced to leave. But we will talk about all this later.

It's comforting to see how feminism is gaining strength and space, taking on voice and body, how we are creating a fabric and building a house where we, all women, can dialogue and shelter. Growing together is easier when one has a place where she can recognize herself and feel protected, knowing that behind her there are more hands and voices that will support her and help her continue on the road ahead.

Understanding the substrate, it would be interesting to see what we can demand of ourselves and what we cannot. We can't demand that the feminisim happening in the cities move at the same pace in our towns. Urban women have to look at their rural sisters differently, begin to really get to know them, outside the Sunday images and news articles. Give them space and a platform, shake hands with them. Recognize them. Because that's how we were able to take to the streets on March 8. Safe, recognized, strong, accompanied. And someday rural women will be able to consider going on strike like women in the cities and to carry out their demands, having the necessary and equal recognition that has been achieved in the cities.

Sometimes it's important to look back. Think about that moment when something ignites: an idea or a simple passage you've read that wakes you up and makes you see things differently. That makes you rethink reality, exercise self-criticism. And most of the time that stimulus that makes things change comes from the outside. I remember the day I was working on an article that we wrote in the Department of Livestock Ecology at the University of Córdoba. I had just finished my degree. We were preparing a publication on the figure of the woman in the rural community. At that time, the word *feminism* wasn't something we heard every-day. In my college I took part in the meetings protesting the Bologna Plan, but there was not a single feminist group or any assemblies about feminism. The germ was there, but the seed hadn't yet begun to grow. In fact, in the same college, where most of the veterinary students were women, we didn't talk about it; we didn't think about why most of our professors were men. I remember that day very well because it was also one of the first sparks that made me wake up, realize that I needed feminism in my life. The data were as follows:

According to data from the INE labour force survey, in 2013 the percentage of women employed in the "livestock, forestry, and fishing" sector was 2.2 percent of the total number of women officially employed in rural Spain.

Only 2.2 percent? I was speechless. I think I started to look for more articles to cross-check the information. I felt like I'd discovered a mistake. No, this couldn't be correct data. 2.2 percent. An insignificant figure, coming close to nothing.

Which country was the one I knew, which I moved around in, and which was the one reflected in those statistics? Where were all those women who have left (and continue to leave) their lives and hands in the fields? Would my grandmother make up part of that 2.2 percent, with her little garden, her chickens, her scales and canning jars, selling her vegetables at symbolic prices to her neighbors? And my mother? Would they appear there, in such an absurd little number? Would such a precise number take into account the cold and the hours my mother spent working as a child among the olive trees on the mountainside helping my grandfather harvest the olives? What about the women livestock producers I knew and worked with? Where were they? How could only 2.2 percent cover all the women working in the rural environment?

Out of these questions everything started. I started looking for these women, wanting to know about them. I tried to be more aware, to be consistent in my day-to-day life. I started to incorporate the word *feminism*, which I hardly heard in my circles and which, until then, I was almost indifferent to. I stopped having misgivings about saying out loud that I was a feminist. It was time to wake up from my lethargy and get started.

I haven't turned thirty yet. I live by myself. I don't have children. My day-to-day life develops and grows in the rural environment: my work doesn't understand schedules or closed geographical spaces. I know that I am young now and I can do this. I don't have kids waiting for me when I leave work, I can go days without sleeping in my own home, traveling thousands of miles without any problem. I love my work, but I know that now is the time I can do it. What will happen the day I decide to become a mother? My work as a field veterinarian is all-encompassing. I write at night, some afternoons I have free, and, most of all, on the weekends. What I mean to say is, I give up my free time most of the time to devote myself to the other job that makes me happy and that's always in my head: writing. But the reality is that I write tired. My working "cultural" self suffers from the schedules of my job as a field veterinarian. I usually get up between five and six in the morning Monday through Friday; most of the days I go out in the field I don't know what time I'll be back, and when it's time to write, I'm too tired to actually do it.

On the other hand, my writing wouldn't exist nor would it be understood without my fieldwork, which occupies so much of my life's space and physical and emotional effort. I have to admit that I'm lucky; sometimes I feel privileged to be able to write in a world where media trends are dictated from offices that are always in big cities. I write from the margins and I have a voice and space to defend what I do and what I believe in, unlike most rural women.

There are difficult days: my writer self wants to give up, drop off to sleep, just sleep. Then, when I read the news, I feel like I have to write, to tell, to make way for other voices, to narrate, to give space, because I can't find the world I move and work in acknowledged by the media. Until very recently, when people wrote about rural women in the news, they used photographs of Indian women working in the fields, in most cases with crops we don't even have in our country. I didn't see one woman I could recognize. Where were they? Why this lack of interest in the hands that care for and work in our rural environment? How could anyone think that such a distant image was more representative than any of those already existing in our nearest territory?

And if I, a woman who works in the rural environment, don't feel recognized, how are these women going to feel?

A few months ago, an interview I gave to the newspaper *El Mundo* about *Field Notebook*, my book of poems, was published under the headline without women, there would be no rural community. I thought it was quite accurate. Because it couldn't be more true and I couldn't agree more with that sentence. A few days went by and I wanted to read comments about the interview on social media. And once again a world appeared that didn't correspond to the one I encountered every day. Many of the comments, most of them written by men, ridiculed the headline. They laughed at it. According to them, women have never worked in the fields, nor have they soiled their hands as much as men. According to them, I'd never stepped foot in a field in my life and, of course, I had no idea what it was like to work in rural areas.

So who's wearing the blindfold?

Women continue to be invisble even though they are there. They work with men and they don't own the land.

They don't make decisions. But every day they work. "They have time" for everything. They call them *all-terrain women* as if it were some kind of praise when it should be admonished and considered a bad thing for a woman to be available for everything and everyone always. Because they get their children ready for school, cook, clean the house, go down to the garden and take care of the chickens, take care of their loved ones (the living and the dead), they never finish that infinite list of household chores and they still "have time." Time for the men, of course. Because after those household chores they go to the fields to help their husband, their father, or their brother with those daily chores, without even having any say in the decision-making or receiving anything in return, and, of course, let's not even talk about shared ownership or having an employment contract. And careful, I'm talking about all the women in our towns. And I'm not referring to those who work alone as livestock producers and farmers and little by little, in a world where men have always been and to a certain extent continue to be in charge, they are making themselves seen and staking claim to their rightful place. They're conscious of all this denial and abuse. I'm talking about *ellas*: about women like my grandmother or like my mother. About all those women I come across when I go to my hometown, those I never recognize but who recognize me. "The granddaughter of Carmen *la gordita*, the woman veterinarian. Go on, give your grandmother a kiss, and one to your mother." Those who always ask about you, about your family. They are happy to see you and that you have a job, that you are an independent woman, that you don't need anyone else to live your life, but then they go on as if nothing happened, *running their errands*, and go back to life as normal all over again.

How can we expose this reality that has no place in the reported statistics, that isn't reflected as it really is anywhere? How can we report that? How can we narrate this unequal dedication between domestic work and care for others? How do we recognize this double workday for the woman in a system where both men and women contribute to the workforce but in most cases it is the men who possess the power to make decisions and determine the outcome of family production. How can we become a spokesperson and support system for *ellas*? How can we claim a feminism for the rural community?

"Silence is a luxury we cannot afford," Chimamanda Ngozi Adichie wrote. And I couldn't agree more. Even if we have our doubts, even if we feel insecure. Even if we're afraid. We have to speak out, raise our voices, write. And I know that the rural community and its women don't need a literature to rescue them, but one that speaks for them. One that is honest and sincere, giving real space to its protagonists. One that doesn't look over their shoulders, doesn't judge or demand, that lets them make mistakes, as we all do, so they can finally tell and write their own story for once. Because we cannot remain silent. Because we need a feminism that is every woman's and for every woman, that overcomes the geographical divide, that dares to leave the big city centers, and that is valid for those who have a voice and can raise it, but especially for those who have a voice and think that theirs is not worth listening to.

A feminism of sisters and land.

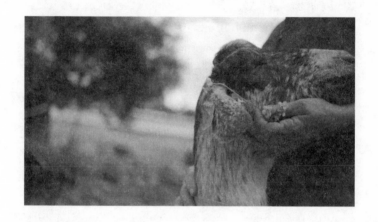

CHAPTER 3

The Caring Hand

Others have labored, and you have benefited from
their labor.

—JOHN 4:38

There's a story told by the writer Jenny Diski in her book
What I Don't Know About Animals that I have carried with
me since I first read it. She recounts that, as a child, she constantly complained about the wool vests her mother forced
her to wear. They were very itchy, and she couldn't stand
them. Her mother always responded the same way. Diski
had to stop her crying and moaning because the garments
she was wearing were made from the finest wool that could
be found in Brussels.

Before telling us this story from her childhood, the writer
draws on previous literature and helps us understand the
concept of *domesticity*. This term, coined by American his-

tory professor Richard W. Bulliet, refers to the "set of social, economic, and intellectual traits that characterize all those communities whose members consider daily contact with animals (with the exception of their pets) as a normal part of their lives."

Diski, recalling her reaction and the subsequent rejoinder from her mother, who emigrated with her parents from the shtetl to England, stated emphatically that she had become a postdomestic subject. Her mother was a subject without any relationship or regular contact with animals. A subject who had completely erased the animals and the environment they inhabit without any regard.

It's not that Diski's mother didn't know what native breed the wool she'd bought came from or which geographic designation those sheep were from that made the wool possible. Where that flock had been raised. Or what the production system was like. Or the factors that gave the product such quality and value to make it the best wool in a city.

It's not that Diski's mother didn't know anything. It's just that she completely ignored it. It's something that didn't exist in her narrative. For her, sheep did not exist, nor did the shepherd or the person who sheared the sheep and treated their wool. For Diski's mother the countryside did not exist. There's no other possibility. By using such an unequivocal statement with her daughter, the rural environment and its inhabitants have no chance of existing. Because they aren't contemplated. They aren't taken into consideration. They don't matter.

This anecdote serves as a way to talk about our rural environment and the rural women who inhabit it. And by *ellas* I'm not referring exclusively to those women who work in the country as livestock producers, farmers, shepherds, or day laborers, but to all those who live in towns throughout our territory. If we can imagine that a large part of the society who live in cities have become postdomestic subjects, for whom the countryside is neither part of nor is thought about in their daily lives, how are they not going to ignore its inhabitants?

We live in a centralist country. Madrid is in charge. The big cities are the decision makers. The ones that set the guidelines, the pace. Sometimes it seems that life and what is important only happen in these nuclei. The rest is always in the background, unimportant, as if it required little. As if its inhabitants had nothing to say.

And if rural areas are largely forgotten, what about the women who live there? Where do they fit in? How can they be considered if they aren't contemplated or taken into account even in the place where they live?

The answer is that rural women are doubly discriminated against. Doubly overlooked. Doubly forgotten. First because of their gender but also because of where they live and work.

We have internalized this ignorance toward our margins, toward the hands that care for them, and toward all the food they produce. This gap between the rural environment and the cities has been grafted onto us. We see it as something normal. We don't ask, we don't question, we don't provide our own account. We don't want to know.

It's true that, in recent times, consumers have started to think twice before deciding what to put in their shopping cart. We are hypnotized by the *eco* and the *organic*, although most of the time we don't turn the food package over to read its label.

Do we wonder where this food comes from?

Has it been produced in our country?

If not, do we question how many miles it has traveled to get to that supermarket shelf?

What about production systems?

Do we know how to differentiate food that comes from

an industrial system? If that meat or that milk or that cheese comes from extensive or intensive livestock farming?

What animals does our food come from? Indigenous breeds? Breeds in danger of extinction?

What about the land?

Monoculture? Polyculture?

Industrial or family farming?

What seeds have been used? What production systems?

The caring hand?

Do we wonder about the people who make our food possible? About their history?

About their working conditions?

Do we stop to think about what it means to have this food at our fingertips?

This is what happens with our food. We live in cities where practically none of what we consume is produced. We need others to do the work, to cultivate, to raise the animals; we need others, in the end, to produce so that we can feed ourselves.

It's true.

We take the food off the shelves and just throw it into the

shopping cart. As if what our hands just dropped had been made right there, in the supermarket, as if it came out of nowhere, without a journey or any history behind it.

We live at the expense of our margins. They are invisible. The cities do not hear their voice, let alone consider that they have one. They do not exist on their own per se. We believe and take for granted that everything that is great and new happens in the city.

Forgive me if I insist:

The rural environment and the women who inhabit it are the great unknowns of the territory.

And it's not because these women have no voice or nothing to say. They do, like every other woman. What happens is that they don't occupy the big platforms, nor do they have the *altavoces* that, coincidentally, are always in the same places, in the big cities.

There's not just one type of rural woman. The rural community is diverse and does not have a single face and voice. The rural community is a multitude. We have many stories to rescue and bring out of the shadows.

> Every day it becomes clearer to me. *Juntas, mejor:* women together are better off.

In a world in which the individual and the immediate are

more and more important every day, it is a necessary and fundamental exercise to turn our gaze upon our margins. It's strange that, in our cities, every day more and more collectives with the goal of creating community emerge and grow. They are characterized by sisterhood, the creation of bonds with the people who form the group, who seek, after all, an exchange of knowledge or assistance. Ultimately, a kind of care. There's also a growing concern in cities to make them sustainable and green. We are worried about pollution, climate change, what we eat. We are afraid of and harmed by solitude. We don't want indifferent cities; we want communities.

Why do we forget our roots?

Why do we forget where we come from?

Why not look at our towns?

A few months ago I read that an initiative called "La escalera," The Stairway, had been started in Madrid. It invites neighbors to get to know others in the building by putting stickers on their mailboxes. I felt a mixture of tenderness and amusement. I started to laugh. I kept imagining the stickers, the neighbors reading them, starting to greet each other after sticking a little piece of paper on their mailbox.

"Now, I can actually knock on the second-floor neighbor's door to see how she's doing. Now someone can pick up my mail, water my plants, keep an eye on my apartment when I'm away or on vacation."

In my head, I kept imagining everyday situations resulting from a sticker on a mailbox. And of course I kept laughing about it.

Because I was thinking of my grandmothers and all the women in towns around the country. In their homes. With their doors open, their entryways always lit. One attentive to the other, taking care of each other. Crossing the street with their warm pots of food, with baskets full of eggs and vegetables, with bread under their arms. Sharing. No need for mailboxes or stickers. There's no need for anyone to think that something that is ultimately so basic and that we carry so deep inside us is original and innovative: affection and care for those around us. Attachment and care. Community and its ties.

I've always thought that what is truly radical and innovative happens at our margins. In our rural areas. In our towns. New bonds, networks that are created, groundbreaking projects, wonderful ideas, associations, collectives…and the ones behind all these initiatives, in most cases, are women.

Women united claiming their rights and making their voices heard. Occupying their rightful places, arriving little by little and, at last, to their livelihood. Taking over the space that was theirs and had always been taken away from them.

Women of land, wind, and livestock.

This is how the extensive livestock producers and shepherds in Ganaderas en Red, the Women's Ranchers Network, like to see themselves. A group of women from different towns around the territory who walk together and fight beside each other for what is theirs. They claim their space as women in the livestock industry, where the man has always been the visible one and who made his voice heard. Women, in livestock production, have always been present, although many people do not want to see their presence, preferring to omit it. Like the women shepherds, women fed up with the idealization of a solitary woman in the countryside resting happily while her animals graze. Also together, hand in hand, they talk and they confront the bureaucracy that makes their task more difficult every day and gets in the way of their work and production methods.

They work together and keep raising their voices for

shared ownership. Because although we live in a time of feminism and in a society in which equality is constantly being demanded, women in our rural environment have always been there, working in the fields, a task that has been chained, as an extension, to all the household chores they already perform. An unfair allocation of the productive role that is always inherent, as such, in the family. Their work with their partners in the fields—I write "work" and not "help" because I am tired of perpetuating this inequality— has never been valued as such and has always appeared reduced, as if it were meaningless, to the category of "family help." This is a reality in the rural world, one full of inequality and, of course, where women are invisible. As the man is the only proprietor, he is also the only face and voice society sees and hears. In the absence of shared land ownership, women still do not exist, in an environment full of harmful consequences for them, and for the society we live in, perpetuating patriarchal values and systems and enabling the rural community to continue to be entirely masculine.

But these women don't only make themselves visible and bring to the table their role as workers in rural areas: shepherds and extensive livestock producers. They go beyond that. They speak openly about all the times they have been left alone at home taking care of their family and their animals, those endless hours devoted to care and house-work. They bring to light the self-imposed standards and the guilt they feel with the work they always carry on their shoulders. Because it's difficult for rurul women to take off that backpack they've been forced to wear from an early age. To be all-terrain women, to be able to handle every-thing, to always be aware and attentive to everything and everyone. We cannot turn this sacrifice and this inequality into a virtue. Our rural women are women like any other, and they need the same as everyone else: to put an end to their constant discrimination and lack of visibility.

As women, they also fight for their communities. Con-nectivity, basic services, education, health care, culture. At what point did we allow our towns and their inhabitants not to have the same rights as the inhabitants of our cities? Why do we continue to perpetuate this discrimination against rural areas and their inhabitants, exacerbating the inequal-ity suffered by their women?

I am not the daughter of, the sister of, the wife of.

How to make the work of rural women visible? How to get rid of that one-dimensional and lifeless postcard where we're framed for contemplation?

The Catalunya Ramaderes are very clear about this: they

will not be silent anymore. This group of women who have come together in Catalonia are an example to follow. Their Twitter bio is a manifesto in itself:

> We are women, we are extensive livestock producers, we are shepherds, we are mothers, we are companions and we are united.

It may seem silly, but social networks are a perfect tool to show the true face of the rural environment and those who work in it. I want to reiterate this a lot because those of us who work in the country can speak out and talk about it; we can have that *altavoz* and that platform that have been denied to us so many times. And I still find it funny that so many people are scandalized by the fact that rural people, especially women, have access to these tools and report on their daily lives. I remember one day I tweeted about how many hours I'd worked among the goats and a user replied to me saying how little work I had and that I wasn't really from the country if I had time to use Twitter. This is the level I'm talking about. And this is unfortunately the image we have of those who work in the country, people without any time or interest enough to talk about themselves.

The dissemination work the Ramaderes do seems essential to me. A few photos of their hands, vindicating themselves, because their hands, even if they are small or thin, even if they are women's hands, are used for work, for milking, for plowing. They don't need a man's hands. These women can do it. The Ramaderes also have an Instagram account. They post pictures of their animals grazing because extensive livestock production and pastorage are a sign of their identity. With slogans like "No shepherdess, no revolution," "Pasture is culture," and "I am not the daughter of, the sister of, the wife of," they make it very clear what their struggle and their daily work is all about. They intermingle their photographs and ideas with quotes from literature written by women. They are openly feminists and are not afraid to point fingers; they know that without them there will be no rural community. They're tired of being the ones in charge of their flocks and still being asked about their husbands. Tired of being framed in that postcard of a beautiful bucolic shepherdess, always wearing a straw hat, asleep while her sheep run around happily. They're tired of how the administration mistreats them and the obstacles they face when marketing their products. Tired of not being included, of being ignored, of being just one more element in the landscape without voice or vote. They have found that the best way to spread their message and make themselves known is through social media. Here are the women who write, who speak out, who care, who narrate their experiences.

> "In Europe, only 12 percent of the land is held by women, compared to 61 percent controlled by men."

When you visit the webpage for FADEMUR, the Federation of Rural Women's Associations of Spain, this is the headline you run into. Like the Catalunya Ramaderes, they use social media to make themselves heard. And since they're on Twitter themselves, they don't want it to rain coffee in the fields, like in the song by Juan Luis Guerra; they want something tangible, they want real action. They want equality. They're immersed in one of the open fronts most in need of change for rural women: *la política agraria común*, the CAP, the common agricultural policy. The policy that, at the end of the day, has the biggest budget and impact on our lives, from when we wake up to when we go to bed, and what we eat for breakfast, lunch, and dinner. The policy that manages the land and those who work on it, but doesn't take rural women into account. The policy that allows for labor exploitation because it remains a mechanism that allows for very low origination prices and large profits along the supply chain through subsidies to large landowners and producers. The policy that expels small, higher-quality producers from the market, those who have better environmental practices, those protecting the country. The policy that hinders land access and never takes into account the word *woman*.

It's imperative that the CAP finally implement a gender perspective once and for all. Urgent and necessary. As Teresa López, the president of FADEMUR, claims, the only thing femine about the CAP is its determining article in Spanish. Its activity is not only important for the inhabitants of rural areas, but also for those who live in the cities. Maintaining our ecosystems and stopping our towns from emptying out once and for all depends on it.

It's obvious that women play a fundamental role in rural areas and that a gender-sensitive agricultural policy is crucial in these places, and that the struggle of women has allowed them to regain their space and raise their voices without fear. Because they are united, because they recognize each other and fight together for their rights and march toward equality.

But what about the women who are still in the shadows?

Our fields are filled with migrant women who are victims of abuse and exploitation. The strawberries we eat are tainted with machismo, harassment, and inequality. Anyone who dares to look under the surface and wants to get closer to the reality of our rural environment will find women working without voice or vote. That cases like those of the seasonal workers in Huelva continue to happen is an atrocious sign of our times. And it's not something new in this land. It took two German journalists, Pascale Müller and Stefania Prandi, to expose what is happening in our fields through a foreign media source. On April 30, they published the story of Kalima, a worker in the strawberry fields who ran away from the man who raped her, her supervisor at work.

It is understood, it is known, but people are silent.

Rural feminism has to protect every woman. Not only women who have managed to get a piece of land or their own flock. Not only women who defend extensive livestock production and other forms of production that respect the

land and its animals. Not only the women who live in cities and identify with ecofeminism, thus weaving more ties
between women, feminism, nature, and ecology. Not only
the women who work in the rural environment on their own
and can speak out and make their demands without being
singled out. We need a rural feminism in which everyone
feels accompanied, in which everyone can help each other
and not feel inferior to each other. We need a rural feminism
that also considers the women who work in those intensive
systems of production—think about strawberries or green-
houses, slaughterhouses, and production chains—who are
often migrant women, without contracts or rights. Who sup-
ports them? Who reaches out to them? Who points the finger
at the culprits without these women becoming the victims?

We must think about the hands that care for and work the
land. When consuming, when traveling, when walking in the
countryside. We must ask ourselves, deconstruct ourselves
again and again. Take nothing for granted. Don't stay on the
surface. Don't think of rural women as mere elements.

We must be aware that we cannot pretend to address the
problem of depopulation in our country by pointing at us,
the women, over and over again. Because we aren't ves-
sels. We aren't an element reduced to the repopulation of

the territory. We want to have the same opportunities, the same rights. We want to be able to choose what neither our grandmothers nor our mothers could choose. To stay or to go. But to have that decision, to have the choice. To have a horizon that opens in front of us and to be the ones to do the telling and the ones who decide. To have access to services and opportunities, without having to abandon the town and go to the city. Never to feel obligated to do anything ever again. Not to return to that painful state of not having a choice, of remaining again and again in that state of resignation. We want a rural environment that is feminist, a land replete with equality and opportunities for the girls of the future, whether or not they are our daughters.

Time goes by and the answer to the following question I asked myself one day while driving, after hearing the story of one of my female livestock producers, is becoming clearer and clearer to me:

> What if the depopulation problem began because of the lack of attention and the constant discrimination against all the women in our towns?

The answer is so obvious it hurts. In every woman's hands, and not only in those of rural women, lies the solution. And although they are the ones who have started projects to keep the rural environment and its inhabitants from dying, we must all get involved so that all women count and are visible.

To achieve a sustainable rural community, one that is both equitable and egalitarian, soon.

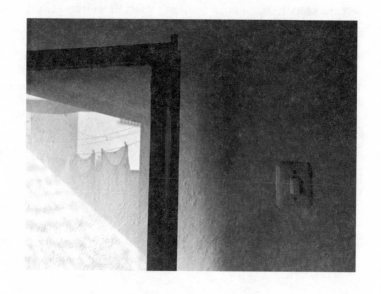

CHAPTER 4

The Emptied Spain

Landscapes can be deceptive.

Sometimes a landscape seems to be less a setting for the life of its inhabitants than a curtain behind which their struggles, achievements, and accidents take place.

For those who, with the inhabitants, are behind the curtain, landmarks are no longer only geographic but also biographical and personal.

—JOHN BERGER

It's difficult to change your way of looking when something you think you know is so profoundly rooted and internalized, stuck deep inside, embedded. And when the outside observer does not step on the same ground or belong to the same stratum as those he's looking at and wants to write about.

Our rural community is so corseted that, whenever it has been written about, the narrative ends up becoming a monologue from the city that we never question.

While I was working with the Galician writer Luz Pichel on a talk on the rural accent at Museum of Contemporary Art at Castilla and León, she uncovered a 1941 black-and-white film titled *O carro e o home*. In it, a voice tells us about the Galician countryside and its inhabitants through the life of a cart. The narrator speaks to us poetically, as if singing a song of praise, about the daily life of the peasants, their tasks, their movements, their life. But the common thread is the cart. From the moment it is built until its last days, defeated, broken, useless, hanging in the patio of a house, a kind of keepsake.

At first glance, the film seems to be made with the best intentions. It helps us understand life in the Galician countryside, its struggles, its customs, its inhabitants. It seems to break from the postcard of the rural environment we have assimilated. Perhaps it was made with an informative purpose, as a way to preserve, as if the ones who made it were the guardians of some seeds on the verge of extinction. To safeguard part of the history of a country, part of the relationship between a territory and its inhabitants.

Throughout the film, the peasants look at the camera, smile. We see strong men and women, working as if they were dancing, with no visible signs of effort or fatigue. Everything looks like a celebration. Work is a game, something unimportant, something that happens and makes the community happy. There's no room for words like *sweat* and *sacrifice*. The children also join in the work, as if there were nothing unusual about that, as if the decision to want to freeze that image of children wearing smocks because they are too poor to wear diapers had no value in itself.

The narrator's voice does not belong to any of the peasants who appear in the film. He speaks in Galician, but anyone who listens to him for a while soon realizes that the narrator is not speaking in his mother tongue. He's not from there; he doesn't belong to the tribe.

And it's this foreign voice that continues to describe the peasants until the end of the film. Not once do we hear their voice portrayed. They're reduced to bodies that work the land, bodies that belong to a space and a context delimited by the narrator.

We could not recover the voice of these peasants because it was never recorded. All we have left is the image. The inscribed postcard from an outsider, constructed out of clear instructions on how to portray the margins. The peasants' voices are taken away, denied, silenced. They are not the ones to tell their own story. Once again, it takes someone from the outside to come in and describe them, enclose them in a rectangle and address their history, their own language, their existence, the very life they lead.

For everyone else, for all those who live in cities, the rural workers are the ones who have nothing to say. Their voices are trapped in the image, frozen, and fade away and will never reach the ears of the spectator. The peasants become mere objects of contemplation. They become one more unimportant piece used to idealize the rural community, to turn it into fiction.

That is why it is essential to ask ourselves again and again about our rural environment:

Who is telling the story about our margins?

Who are the ones writing about our rural community?

And despite the fact that it is always the same people who write about us, through their work, be it images, books, articles, or simple commentaries, the light continues to seep in because there are fragments, breaks in the landscape, fissures.

It is through these little crannies where the light continues to pass, where we can learn to find and read what no longer exists, what no longer matters, what is no longer recounted in an intentional way.

O carro e o home is a perfect exercise to train our sight, to rescue everything that is not seen. If we pay a little more attention, if we put aside the omnipotent voice of the narrator, we will find elements that, although they were always there, we had not noticed at first glance: Community work, native breeds that today no longer exist or are on the verge of extinction, sustainable production methods such as family farming and extensive livestock production, vocations that are no longer visible, that are relegated, at best, to those small museums in some towns that are always closed. Links between the inhabitants. Group. Community. Words. Language.

In the end, culture.

But what happens when a group of people is made to feel inferior because they belong to a certain social class or place and their entire identity is taken away from them?

What happens when a model of life is imposed on a

group? When their language is taken away? Their links? Their ways of life?

How can you be proud of your roots if you've been taught since the time you can first remember that the only possible way to get ahead is to leave?

How can you recognize yourself if the mirror in front of you belongs to someone else who speaks another language and whose hands look different than yours?

How can you appreciate what surrounds you and consider it your own if you are already born inferior, if the system itself despises your way of life?

Our grandmothers wear it on their foreheads. Like so many older people in our towns. Feeling ashamed of where they come from. Hiding their hands in the pockets of their coats when someone from outside the community arrives. Preferring silence over their own voice. Working tirelessly so their children can leave. Accepting as normal everything that was taken from them and turned them into second-class citizens. Accepting that these women are not the ones who decide what we need. Seeing as normal that someone from outside always comes in to construct the story, deciding what we want, what we need, what we feel. Even weaving our own aspirations.

Yes, they idealize us. But we are inferior. Because they won't let us speak.

They decide to render us mute. That our voice won't be heard. That our mouth and our hands become useless elements, without words to accompany their own movements. They deny our own language the light and nourishment it needs.

They don't let us speak; they don't let us decide.

The peasant's mark on the forehead. The stain of being from a small town. The painful association of the rural community with terms like *redneck*, *ignorant*, *brute*, *simple*, *bumpkin*, *hick*, *inferior.*

Inferiority is stuck deep inside.

One day, when I finished working with one of the livestock producers in the association I work for, I walked around the barn to wash my hands in a basin in the farmyard. When I looked up I saw a pile of rubble resting against the plaster wall in front of me. I couldn't help moving closer. Among the broken barrels, bricks, and sacks, I saw the remains of a cart. That component that gave structure to life in the countryside in the film and was a link between the person, the animal, and the environment was just another piece of garbage here. In that farmyard the cart didn't end its days resting against the wall, after a life of support and assistance: it doesn't become a memory, something to be proud of. The next thing I knew, I was asking my colleague about the wagon. He laughed. He didn't understand how I could feel such an attraction for something so old, something he had always seen like that, since he was little, some meaningless wood scraps, disassembled, discarded, ridiculous, absurd, useless. I thought about the hands that at some point carved the wood and fitted it together. About the voice that would call the mule that would pull the wagon. I wanted to know who had made the cart. Maybe his grandparents? He didn't know how to respond. Those pieces of wood were just one more element in his workplace, as if a consequence of the environment. All he knew was that they were very old, that it never crossed his mind to think about their age. And he had no one to ask about it. The wagon meant nothing to him because he had grown up with it being there. And with that acceptance of the inferior thing, both his history and that of his ancestors, the entire genealogy of the land we walked on was erased in one stroke. It ceased to exist and have any value. It evaporated. It disappeared.

How can we begin to write about what is ours if we've been taught to never place any importance on it?

How can we redefine the word *culture* in the rural community if we've never considered the rural community to be cultured?

How do we learn to look inside the fissures?

It's up to us, our generation, to remove that mark from our people. It's up to us not to be ashamed of our roots or our blemishes. It's up to us to speak out. We can't allow them to take away our voice and let others come once again to tell us our own stories. It's up to us to point, to make people see, to change the light on the postcard so that the viewer doesn't see it the same old way, so that the observer doesn't fictionalize us again.

We live in a time when the rural environment always appears in the news media and on social networks. There isn't a literary supplement or magazine that doesn't dedicate at least part of its contents to the countryside and its inhabitants. They talk about depopulation, about communities being abandoned and elderly people dying alone. Rural-themed books tell us about the voices that are dying out. And it always has to be someone who comes from the city to tell their story, to capture their lives on paper so that they don't disappear in vain. Summer arrives and, with the heat, the newspaper columns fill with nostalgia for childhoods spent in our towns, for bike rides, for evenings in the town plazas with the neighbors. But also for towns as a way to escape, as an oasis for rest and flight from the cities. As the perfect place to disconnect and be apart from the world. Similar to that image of a Walden-like cabin in the middle of nowhere, off the grid and out of range, the perfect escape from the world that is drowning us. The rural environment is in fashion.

But how?

Again:

Who tells the story?

What comes to light and what remains hidden in the shadows?

In most cases we find that those who write about our rural environment are men. Men without any connection to the community, men who do not work in it. Men who live in the big cities and go to the country on the weekend so they can write about it. Men who travel miles and miles to write about us. Men who, though it may not be their intention, are taking away our voice. They are letting us not decide. They reduce us to what they want to say about us. They take it for granted that we have neither voice nor space, and that we are incapable of telling our own stories.

Gentlemen, no offense. I don't want to require that only those who are from the country can write about the country. But it's time for you to understand that the same people have always written about our regions and our towns. That we don't need you to give us our own voice. We already have it. We know how to speak, write, narrate. We have a community full of stories, words, lives, seeds, paths, animals, trees, connections, people. We don't want a literature that labels us with someone else's words, or that it is this literature that decides what we are called while we, women, are learning not to be ashamed of our roots and our land. We don't want a narrative that calls us *farmers*. That labels us. We don't want more newspaper columns full of nostalgia for dying towns. We, rural women, are tired of living in Sunday news articles. Tired of being reduced to characters in *The Holy Innocents.* Saddened to become the coffins you bury inside that terrain you say is empty. Bored with you framing us only in scenes of hunger, pain, and misery.

We're sick of always seeing ourselves in that same flat, boring postcard because we're nothing like that. Because our day-to-day life, our existence, is nothing like that.

We are not the emptied Spain.

We are an extensive territory full of life. Of people, of stories, of vocations, of communities.

We are women shepherds, day laborers, agriculturists, mule drivers, olive growers, livestock producers. We are the caring hand that has made it possible for the places that are now considered national and natural parks in this country to be such. Through the action of the shepherds and their flocks. Through extensive livestock production. Because of so many men and women who worked in the country and created a unique and special bond between animal, person, and environment. And those of us who work on the land are only one part of the diversity of the rural environment.

The rural environment and its inhabitants do not need to be rescued by any literature. They need to be recognized at last, to occupy their own space and regain their voice. More than ever, they need their problems and needs to be truly addressed. Our towns are dying and what we need most are real solutions, uniform policies, emergency measures, public awareness. They need the same services that are available to our sisters and brothers in the cities. There's no need for more stories and literature if they always come from the same people. The rural community doesn't need paternalism or romanticism, or headlines that continue to define its members as the rough men and women who populate our countryside.

The rural community wants a hand to reach out to it with assistance; it doesn't want to be used once again as a place for recreation or scandal. Like a beautiful oasis to turn into fiction.

The countryside doesn't need cities to make it more attractive. It already is. It needs recognition and honesty. For those who are looking at it to really learn how to understand it, without already prejudged images or filters.

Many of our grandmothers and grandfathers never held their heads high because they were from a village. They expected to learn from outsiders. They were always the invisible, the silent, the illiterate ones. Always letting others come to construct our story for us.

Now it's our turn to create our narrative. To begin to draw our genealogy. One that considers us, one that goes beyond the simple, flat image. One that embraces our connections, our animals, our trees, our paths. One that knows about care and other forms of sustainable production. One that wants to learn our songs and our languages. One that neither disdains us nor dictates. One that looks, inquires, and questions. A narrative that steps forward, that gets dirt on its hands and is not ashamed.

And despite the fact that we finally began to occupy the spaces that belonged to us, which we pointed out, and in the end we did not remain silent, sometimes I think we arrived late.

Like in *O carro e o home*, we have allowed vocations and words to die by not recognizing them as our own. Like our heritage, like our culture. Sometimes my fear returns, like the fear I felt when I didn't recognize my grandfather's voice, when I heard people from the country using words that are unfamiliar, words that in the cities are not heard, and that do not exist there. Many of these words no longer even appear in the the Royal Spanish Academy's Spanish dictionary.

Where will all that knowledge go when the last people who use it and understand it die?

How can we allow part of who we are to die like this? Why do those of us living in the cities not even consider that this belongs to everyone?

Culture.

I go back to the dictionary. Sometimes I'm afraid to go in and see that they have erased the first definition of the word, that they want to eliminate every last trace of the origin of the word *culture*.

First meaning:

> 1. f. cultivation.
> Of the land.

What germinates.
What grows.
What it nourishes.

What makes life possible.

Over and over again.

Again, the blindfold keeping us from looking at the margins.

The time has come for untrembling hands to remove it.

For hands that point to those who would take away their voice.

For hands that write their own story and forget the mark of the peasant on their foreheads.

For hands that care for their rural environment and all that it contains, like those shepherd dogs that vigilantly keep watch, accompanying from a distance, the sheep in their flock that are about to give birth and so stray off on purpose, wander off alone, looking for a distant and quiet place to bring their lambs into the world and make life possible once again.

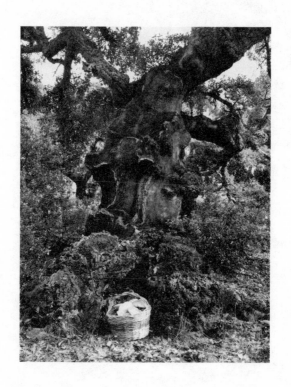

CHAPTER 5

For a Living Rural Community

My whole childhood is the countryside. Shepherds, fields, sky, solitude. In short, simplicity. I am always so surprised when people think that those things in my work come from my own audacities, the audacities of a poet. No. They are authentic details, which many people find odd because it is also odd to approach life with such a simple and so little-practiced attitude: watch and listen....I'm more interested in the people who inhabit the landscape than the landscape itself. I can gaze at a mountain range for a quarter of an hour, but I immediately run to talk to the shepherd or woodcutter in those mountains. Then, when I'm writing, I remember one of these dialogs and the authentic expression of the people emerges. A large archive in my memories of childhood is filled with memories of hearing people talk. It's my poetic memory and I look after that.

—FEDERICO GARCÍA LORCA

Sometimes I feel as if rural people and city dwellers speak a different language. That we don't understand each other. We hear each other, we recognize each other's faces and gestures, but we don't listen to each other. Words remain suspended in the air, but they don't germinate in any substrate. We are both part of a dialogue, but we don't understand each other. As if language widened the distance between the countryside and the city. As if the face-to-face encounter occured on each side, only in front of an opaque mirror that never shows a reflection.

The Basque writer Bernardo Atxaga begins his book *Marks*, in which he writes about the unnamed and unaccounted for dead in the Guernica tragedy, with a beautiful reflection about some inscriptions carved into a rock in a museum in Milan. *Il masso di Bormo* isn't just any stone. The marks on the rock are seven thousand years old. They're unintelligible. There's no way to read them. The idea of a language or a message doesn't exist. They're just marks. Incisions in a stone by someone who wanted to leave a mark there. We don't know why, with what intent, or if they meant anything. But what can't be read or understood reaches us all the same. We can see that unknown language, touch it, try to decipher it. What if it doesn't matter what it says? What if the mark had another purpose beyond causes or intentions?

Atxaga translates: the incisions aren't understood, but they continue pulsing. Because they transmit a message, thousands of years later they manage to bring us a clear and hardly disputable message:

We were here, one day we were alive here.

The mark on the stone, like the opening that indicates but at the same time separates.

I recognize myself in Atxaga's fragment. A rural community that attempts to tell its story, to make its problems known. A territory full of people who don't want to leave and do everything possible so they don't have to. Who wave their arms for help, who point out the absences, who have an impact on what we have to preserve.

But the mark has been made. And those on the outside are now beginning to acknowledge it. They talk about depopulation, lack of resources and services, climate change, nature, conservation..., but they never seem to find the exact language to move beyond the concepts, to move beyond headlines that never fully express and show the true face of our rural environment and its inhabitants.

> What if we need a new language to build bridges between the rural and urban?
>
> What if we all have to once again learn how to name?

Despite my roots, my work, and my intense bond with the rural environment, I too often become that stranger who arrives in a place where they speak a different langauage she doesn't understand. It's especially painful when you realize this is happening to you even with your own family.

At some point it dawned on me that I didn't understand many of the words my family used to talk about their daily lives, or to communicate with me, words I'd heard so many times without paying attention to them. I wasn't familiar with them. I didn't know what they meant. They weren't part of *mi lengua*, my tongue, my language.

This awakening turned into an obsession. I started asking questions and every unfamiliar word suddenly became new to me. I became a little girl again. I took advantage of every moment to point and ask. And not only with my parents, my aunts and uncles, and my grandparents. The pointing hand and the questioning voice also reached the people in the towns where I went to work and the herdswomen and men I spend almost all of my days with.

Part of me still feels guilty.

If I, someone who moves between the country and the city, was beginning to lose my rural tongue, the language of my people, to what extent had it not already disappeared for those who live in the cities?

I tested it out. I began to collect those words like seeds and I put them in a notebook, safeguarded them, held them close, as you do when you gather seeds and you place them on paper to dry them and, once they are ready, save them in little glass jars in the pantry or in the storeroom for the next sowing. That's how the words of my family began to travel from our town to the city and to recognize a new soil to cling to. When I was with my friends, at work or at some literary event, I couldn't help taking out my notebook and tossing out a word or two without revealing the meaning. I threw them out like a farmer sows seeds onto the soil, hoping they would take root, sprout, and bear fruit.

Most of the words I carry to the city are unknown, but they awaken something that can't be named, that we carry inside and that is still there, latent, waiting for the right light to be detected. They rouse from sleep an interest that keeps the language of my family and so many others alive.

And they rescue something else. Unfamiliar words awaken questions of their own, new names, old memories. They rescue the connection and manage to bring a new language to the surface to start cultivating. Words like *fardela*, the backpack or sack shepherds use. Like *galiana*, a trace or smaller path transhumants use. Like *cabellano*, that terrain in the mountains which is flat, with hills and valleys, but gentle ones. Like *empollo*, the first grass that grows in autumn after the first rains. Like *jabardillo*, that group of birds smaller than a flock.

In 2002 *Science* magazine published an article titled "Why Conservationists Should Heed Pokémon." I came to it much later, in September 2017, because the English writer Robert Macfarlane mentioned it in his article "Badger or Bulbasaur—Have Children Lost Touch with Nature?" in the *Guardian*.

The title of the article caught my attention. How to marry nature conservation with something as strange and distant from it as Pokémon? The text showed the results of tests that had been carried out on English children between the ages of four and eleven with different illustrated cards, always without the name of the item shown. The cards showed different elements: trees, insects, birds, animals… and Pokémon. The results were quite disheartening. They recognized 80 percent of the Pokémon. Wildlife less than 50 percent.

But how can we love what we do not know?

How can we protect and preserve what is so unknown and so far away from us?

How many of us know how to recognize a cork oak, an oak, a holm oak, an olive tree, a poplar, a rockrose, or an ash tree?

Do we know which plants we're gathering, the ones we're constantly stepping on?

Do we recognize the animals we see on the side of the road? Do we know their names?

And the birds crisscrossing in front of you? Do we go beyond sparrows, blackbirds, starlings, storks, and swallows?

Do we wonder about them?

What if they're in danger of extinction?

What if this is the last time we see them?

We want a countryside that is alive and green, but do we know how to identify its shepherds? Do we know our trees? Do we know how to name the species that live there? Do we really understand our protected spaces and do we know how to identify, for example, other ways of raising livestock such as extensive livestock production? Do we value those invisible caring hands and the valuable food they produce?

I'm not trying to reduce everything to names. But it's important to learn to name and recognize in order to conserve and nurture. Like children. Go back to that excitement, to those hands always pointing, to that voice that never stops growing and only wants to learn new names and sensations.

Why don't we see more of ourslves in children?

Every time I go back to the country, for work or with my family, I feel like a child again. To the root, the cradle, the lullaby. Each trip back makes me want to soak up more of it. Get involved. Create a network with my people. Involve others in the process. So the network expands and reaches more places.

The rural community needs more than just a language

to survive. But only when we take off our masks, get rid of our prejudices, and sit down at the same table, face to face, without complexes, without paternalism, without contempt or superiority, will we be able to begin to change things. When we free ourselves from what's supposed to be true and begin to question, to lose our shame, to question ourselves. Like when we were children because we wanted to learn and name, we wanted to be part of the new world that was opening before our eyes, to feel like we were part of it and of everything else. When we speak the same language. That's how we can begin to understand each other.

I'm tired of pitting the rural against the urban. We need each other and nothing good comes from confrontation. We must level the playing field on both sides to close a gap that has become too big, too painful.

Everything inside our territory, our rural environment, can't be enclosed in a book. It would be absurd to try to cover the entire countryside with paper. Our countryside, its inhabitants, and elements are an infinite heritage. I don't want this to be an instruction manual so our countryside doesn't die, so our towns don't disappear. I don't want and I can't and I don't believe that this is my mission. I could write lists, manuals, causes, consequences. I could speak in depth about depopulation, ground abandonment, the different models of production, shepherds and animals, ravines and trails, a multitude of stories and seeds that have brought me this far.

But that's not my job.

I'm a simple field veterinarian who is a woman and works in the rural evironment every day. I'm not a woman expert on depopulation, I'm not a woman sociologist, I'm not a woman politician, I'm not a woman specialist, I'm not a woman livestock producer, I'm not a woman farmer, I'm not a woman shepherd, I'm not a woman researcher, I am not.

No one person alone has a solution for anything. We need each other to question ourselves, to change our consumption patterns, our ways of seeing, to want to preserve and not abandon, to stand shoulder to shoulder and not turn our backs. We all have to reach out to each other. It's our job to make a green and sustainable future possible in our towns. Change is at the margins, where there is a tomorrow, where another way of life is possible.

And I, I don't want them to exist only in my memory.

I just want to be an excuse to open up the word and reconstruct the language, the hand that gathers seeds from one side and sprinkles them on another, like those seeds that get caught on the loins of the transhumant animals to germinate thousands and thousands of miles away from their place of origin. Let language, like life, endure and discover a multitude of forms, paths, encounters, and words to continue to hold on, to continue to survive, to, in the end, continue to exist.

I want this book to become a land where we can all settle down and find a common language. A land where we can feel like siblings, where we can recognize each other and look for alternatives and solutions. Only then will we be able to scratch under the surface and talk about depopulation, agroecology, culture, extensive livestock production, food sovereignty, territory.

I want the new words to germinate without fear. Let them propagate. Let them become a river full of life that reflects an image we recognize, close and familiar. An image we want to be part of.

Because, through the word, I feel that my love for and my bond with the rural enviornment reaches further. When I leave behind what I've learned in books. It happens and becomes real, when I let my experience speak. When I allow my writing and my day-to-day life to emerge from what I have lived.

From what is part of me.

This is not only my homeland, nor is it exclusive to the inhabitants of our towns. This country belongs to everyone.

And it has been a homeland full of men and women who have been dying alone, covered with moss and birds, waiting for someone to discover them.

A land that has finally ceased to be ashamed of what it is, that recovers its place and names it, makes itself heard, begins to leave crumbs along the paths so that the rest of us look at the ground and want to follow the trail.

Yes, a homeland full of people who were assumed to be nameless, voiceless. Those with dirty hands, sweat on their foreheads; those with their feet on the ground. Those wearing espadrilles and whistling at their animals, smelling like the countryside, always with an aftertaste of damp earth.

All those who work the land and who in their own way, like those who etched into that stone seven thousand years ago, leave their mark with their hands and their labor. And no matter how much nature does its work and how much oblivion and abandonment want to impose themselves, their marks, their tracks, their footprints will endure.

But you can still recognize us.

You can still understand us.

We are still speaking in the present tense.

A living rural community that stands up and reaches out to you.

A territory full of people who fearlessly tell you:

We are alive and we are here.

PART TWO

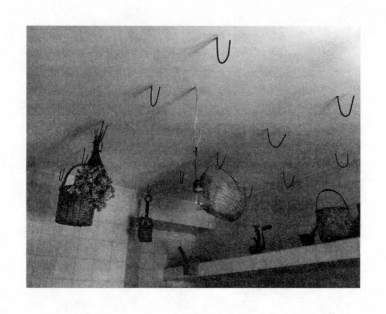

CHAPTER 1

Three Women

As a child I loved a lichen-bitten name.

—SYLVIA PLATH

As she was dying, the mother of the writer Terry Tempest
Williams grabbed her hands and told her she was leaving
her all of her notebooks. The condition: the daughter had
to promise not to open the notebooks until her mother was
gone. Terry recounts this in her book *When Women Were
Birds*. She didn't know her mother wrote anything or that
she had saved all those words on paper. The surprise flooded
her with pain. Suddenly, something had been revealed that
before that moment had been in the shadow, something
unknown and strange. The possibility that her mother was
also writing in her own voice, outside of herself, apart, existing on her own, by herself. When her mother dies, Terry
has the three boxes of notebooks with her. She decides to

open them, read them, take care of them, and she is even more surprised when she discovers that the notebooks are completely empty. No word, no line, no stain whatsoever. There's nothing there.

It is this absence that leads Terry to write her book. To search among the roots of the women in her family. To ask herself again and again what it means to have a voice. For her, opening all those inherited notebooks one after the other and discovering that they were empty was like burying her mother for the second time. A second death, a repeated and open grief that stretched across the blank white pages. Can a color ache? Absence, emptiness, loneliness, the outdoors, snow, weeping. Everything concentrated in insolent white.

My mother's journals are paper tombstones.

And out of nothing the questions start, the steps backward, the explorations. The way back to the mother who is no longer here. Terry wonders about her mother's former life and realizes that she knows nothing. Only one narrative appears and repeats itself over and over again in all the women in her family. Their stories begin to exist when they become mothers. It's only when their children appear that they become visible. Never by themselves, always with their children, behind and beside. These women don't exist on their own, they're not important, as if it were not necessary to speak or do anything before becoming mothers. As if their life and voice are given to them once they have children. Empty paper notebooks, blank, for their children to write in and have their own life and voice while, little by little, the lichen begins to do its work, begins to cover these women. To erase once and for all what was never told or written down.

The lichen has not yet done its job because I haven't forgotten their names yet. I keep them written down, always close to me. But just because I can still name them doesn't mean they're immune to corrosion and oblivion. Two of the three women are still here but I haven't really been aware of them until very recently. Once again, the need for genealogy, to learn to look, to rest in that place in the shade that we believe is invisible and alone. I don't want what happened with the rest of the women in my family to happen to them. I don't know the names of many of these women, where they were born, what they did for a living, what they were like. Meanwhile, the tree branches of the men in my house are more clearly drawn, more defined, less susceptible to the damp moss that ends up making them disappear. I have to admit that this is a self-imposed exercise. An inverse path to my roots. Three women who walked before me and smoothed the path that I am walking on today.

I use the term *the first daughter* a lot to talk about myself, about my situation as a third-generation veterinarian, being the first woman in my family to go into the profession. But it's true that I was the first granddaughter, the first daughter, the first niece. And until recently I didn't realize that by speaking in the first person, always about myself and my circumstances, I was leaving all the other women in my family behind. Recently, a friend told me about something that had happened to her with one of her daughters. She was reading a story to the youngest so she would fall asleep when the little girl started to ask her endless questions about her mother. Then, about her mother's mother, ceaselessly searching for the mothers of the mothers. Suddenly, her daughter falls silent, as if gathering her breath, and she asks: "Mamá, what about the first mother? Who is the first mother of all of us?"

I'm obsessed with stories about connections. Since I was a little girl, I can't help but be attracted to the relationships between animals and their herders, between the herders and the dogs that guard the flock, between trees and the ground where they grow, between birds and the place they choose to build their nest and nurture their young. The same thing happens to me with seeds and their multiple defense and survival mechanisms.

We attach great importance to language. I think of the first word, which we learned and which came out of our inexperienced mouths, trembling, with our own voice, like those mammalian mothers who walk nervously, between instinct and doubt, turning in circles and looking from side to side before lowering themselves and lying on the ground, before the sweet scent of placenta and colostrum comes, before they turn their heads and recognize by smell this first offspring that never stops looking for its mother, stumbling, not yet having enough time to open its mouth and embrace the language. The word *mamá*.

But it's not just voice or language that helps us stand up and keep going. Maybe it's necessary to go to a more earthly, more corporeal, more instinctive aspect. Which has to do with where we come from, where we were born. Because it's not easy to find a narrative, a tale, or a story, a mythology even, where the protagonists and the gods are born from excrement, from some fluid like blood or the maternal liquids that form in the placenta. What we mistakingly consider dirty. This image that we don't name, we don't speak of, belongs to a blurred time that doesn't fit in our childhood memories and our first words, and is irredeemably linked to women. The first word always appears clean, decisive, forceful, but never "stained" with amnios or body. It appears just like that, without genealogy or stains, without blood, without milk.

I think a lot about the first hand that held mine. Of that mammalian geography, warm, invisible, of care and attachment, which has always been there, but which has passed in silence, carrying too many things on its back, reaching out to others, without looking after herself. That hand that helped me grow up without fear of falling or getting dirty, despite the time I've spent not seeing or recognizing it.

Around these connections there is a common image in my childhood that also often occurs in my work, without any warning. It's a mother's rejection of a newborn she knows isn't hers. She pushes it away, hits it with her head, ignores it. She doesn't care if it doesn't eat; she won't allow it to get close to her udders. She acts like this little creature doesn't exist and doesn't matter. There is no adoption or pity for the orphan. The mother doesn't recognize the scent that rises up in the shock of labor when the newborn appears and the bond between mother and offspring is formed. This new member of the flock isn't recognized and can't be part of it. There's no language option. All recognition or belonging is reduced to smell, to instinct. It may also be intuition. This is something that we can't know with certainty. That is why shepherds skin the lambs that die as soon as they are born. And they bind the hide of the one that is no longer living to the orphans. As if it were a cloak, a wrapper, one more chance at life. The orphan's survival depends on the new scent that now embraces it. If the mother recognizes it as belonging to her, she accepts and raises the little one as if it were her own. This is how the bond is born and continues.

I don't know if my mother will leave me notebooks when she dies, but I don't want to wait until she's gone to find out. I don't want it to happen with my grandmother Carmen either. I don't want them to disappear for me to start asking myself questions. My great-great-grandmother Josefa began to exist this year because of a story my father told me on a walk through the countryside while we were talking about cork oaks. They are the three women. Three stories that have existed without me and on their own, but until recently I haven't wanted to look at them. Outside of me and without me they exist. They don't need me for that. It's a mistake we continuously make as children, believing we are the protagonists, the singing voices, the only ones with the right to make everything revolve around us.

Some women are gone and other women are far away.

I do not want these lines by Anna Akhmatova, lines I've taken the liberty of changing the gender in as a small rebellion against the system, to become a maxim for my life, a truth to which I arrived late and could not change. I don't want to have to rely only on the lives of other women, like the orphan wearing the skin of the dead newborn, to feel recognized and supported. I don't want blank white pages, or questions that can never be answered. I want to be that cloak, that shelter for them. I don't know if it will be a relief or if it will be worth anything, but there is something in me, primal, like the scent the mothers need to recognize their lambs, that continuously asks me to do it. Hence the writing.

My paternal great-great-grandmother, my maternal grandmother, and my mother. Not all the women in my family are here, but these three are the ones who still are in one way or another and they are the ones I feel closest to. The women I always carry with me. Let this essay serve as an exercise of justice and recognition for their memory. As a way of not feeling guilty, of redeeming myself for all these years in which they were not part of my narrative or the mirror I wanted to see myself reflected in. Here the first daughter doesn't matter; here the hands, the voices, the caring tell the story. I am who I am only with them; may my writing at least be a refuge. Because I don't know if I will be a mother, or if I will fill drawers and drawers with blank notebooks. I do know that now is the time to look in a different way, to relearn, to change my language and how I step.

Is making a living through writing a blind way to be useful to the species?

This question that Maria Gabriela Llansol wrote in one of her diaries has been haunting me for years. I must admit that I've taken it to heart. Maybe because it was also a way to justify myself, to make sense of my writing. Today, after everything, I finally make sense of it. I might know the answer today.

Friends, sisters, compañeras, yes. I think so. I think we still have time.

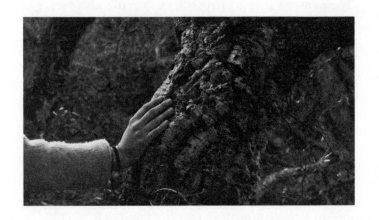

CHAPTER 2

Great-Great-Grandmother: Cork Oak

In 1665, the Englishman Robert Hooke, one of the most important experimental scientists in history, published the book *Micrographia*: a compendium of fifty microscopic and telescopic observations with their corresponding drawings. It is in this book that the word *cell* appears for the first time in history. When studying a sheet of cork oak under the microscope, Hooke discovered that the material was arranged in space in the form of compartments. This arrangement of the cork reminded him of cells, just as the rooms in monasteries are also called.

The first cell described in history is reminiscent of a room. A space demarcated by four walls. A safe place. A place to take refuge, sleep, and pray. A room of one's own, as laid claim to by the writer Virginia Woolf. Although we might take the meaning of the word *cell* to the other extreme, a contrary sensation. Claustrophobia, solitude, confinement. Absolute lack of freedom.

Like so many women, I don't have a room of my own where I write. I write at the same table where I do the paperwork for my veterinary practice in the afternoon, after hours, answering emails, filling out spreadsheets, cleaning up my field notes. I write at the same table where I eat. I write at the same table where my life happens, a demarcated space, flat, without walls to contain it, but leaning against a wall, which becomes the only horizon where I can curl up and write. My life happens at this table because it is the first place I put everything as soon as I get home. The books that arrive, my laptop, my keys, the shopping, my work bag, the clothes I've brought in from the rooftop clothesline, the notes and notebooks scattered across the tabletop along with jottings that never appear later when I need them. Whenever I sit at the table I have to stop and reposition everything that rests on the surface. Everything that's in the way of the task I want to do. This is my cell. This is a cell of my own.

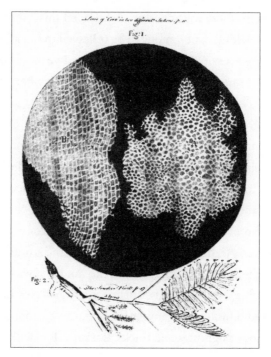

Cork cells

But before I get to the table, before the notes, the cross-outs, and the writing, I need to walk. Go to town, come back. Step where my ancestors did. I need this exercise, as if it were a kind of ceremony to be followed to the letter, an absolute necessity. These past few years I've gone back to doing the same thing that made me so happy when I was a child. Go back to my hometown whenever I can, escape to my family's land. Watch my uncle work with his animals, the mutual understanding he has with his herding dogs, try to help him, soak up everything he tells me and what he doesn't tell me, his gestures and his chores, his dedication to the land. Details that are unimportant until they happen and materialize. Also the days seem shorter when I go out with my father, and he goes on telling me stories about those who inhabited and worked the land. I always come back with a notebook full of plant names, species in Latin and their familiar denominations, feathers, notations in pencil about sightings and tracks. Baskets filled with mushrooms, asparagus bunches, oregano sprigs, cloth bags filled with sloeberries. Walking through the countryside with him isn't limited to just stepping on the ground and contemplation. It is a complete foray into the land and everything on it. Because you learn to look at the landscape in a different way, you begin to see elements that at first do not appear, that do not fit in the first image that takes shape in front of you. You also start to watch where you are stepping, you are more careful where you walk, you have to know how to walk in the country without making noise, disrupting as little as possible the invisible path that you have, without realizing, begun to gestate. You become an attentive observer, expectant of any change that may occur in front of you. A bird song you haven't heard before, the crackle of some nearby twigs, an unexpected encounter with an animal that emerges and makes time stand still in that instant. When your eyes meet, as if that gaze needed the second hand of the watch to stop in order to catch its breath before moving on. As if life from time to time needed a pause to get a running start and continue on.

Last winter, walking one afternoon near the riverbank, my father began to talk about cork oak trees that were dying without remedy, that were falling down, like those elderly people who are fine one day and suddenly suffer a downturn and never recover. Everything becomes an uphill battle. They simply let themselves go. And while he spoke, we kept moving forward. Near a mound of stones beside the little meadow, the ruins of an old shepherd's house appeared as if they were a sign. It was there, a few steps away from the phantom house:

A three-hundred-year-old cork oak. Ash-colored.
Broken.
Its branches fallen.
Overtaken by death.
Quercus suber
From the *Fagaceae* family, those that give sustenance.

Quercus was the Roman name for oaks in general and their wood, and it was also used to designate trees that produce acorns. The origin of the word is Celtic. It means "beautiful tree."

It's imposing to see a tree like this agonizing, dying, beginning to disappear. Because even if the tree splits, turns gray, and lets itself be ravaged by fungi and lichen, life goes on around it. On the ground, on the trunk, on the branches. Birds nest, insects feed, mushrooms take advantage of the organic matter. If any branch remains it will continue to give shade, rest, refuge. Water will nestle in its nooks and crannies. Life always goes on, despite death.

We had to bump into it deliberately to get my father to talk. That day he confessed that he always sits and rests on that tree. That it gives him peace, calm, something he can't describe in exact words but it makes him feel good, something he needs to keep going.

Father and daughter sit down. One leans her back against the tree, the other stays close. They breathe. The daughter gets up, she needs to touch the cork that will never again be harvested from the tree. It will never be separated from the body again; there will be no room for regeneration. What covers it becomes a coffin for the tree itself. The daughter notices the texture in the palm of her hand, tries to intuit what's still inside, the wounds, what is never seen at first sight. The father is silent.

How to know the age of a tree?

The father stands up, uses a stick like a cane which will also serve for pointing. If the cork isn't removed properly, he indicates, the planks of cork get stuck to the neck of the tree, one overlapping the other. Remains of cork adhered to the "male cork," the *bornizo*, the first cutting.

Bornizo, like the first child who doesn't let go, doesn't leave, who prefers to stay. It's the virgin cork, rough, old, the only one that understands and has grown next to the trunk. Like the first cell. The first word. The first scent. The original bark.

The daughter nods. Hesitates. She would rather the father tell her the age. She allows herself to be carried away by the silence. She likes it when her father laughs at her because she doesn't tie her shoelaces properly—*at your age and you still haven't learned*—and bends over to tie them, like when she was a little girl. She knows those days are far away, that the ones where she will be telling her father things, the ones where she will tie his shoes, are closer.

This is how you can tell the age of a cork oak. Touching. Counting one by one the layers of cork that stayed behind like witnesses of the extractions. Cork is stripped every nine years. She counts. She counts and multiplies. This is the way you can work out its age. Without harming it, without having to cut the trunk to get to the growth rings.

But what is removed is also a form of protection for the organism. Thanks to the cork planks, the tree is protected from fire; there's a chance to survive fire. And that casing, which on this tree becomes a kind of casket, is what provides a livelihood where I come from.

Where I come from, cork harvesting is a man's job exclusively. They are the ones who climb the tree, strip the cork, lead the mules, load the cork planks, rest in the shade, and have lunch midmorning. There's no place for women here;

it's not considered, it's not discussed. The work is done in summer, in the July heat, in the company of supervisors and the animals waiting to be loaded down with layers of the tree. It is delicate, meticulous work. There's a rhythm to it. The axes make a songlike sound. The cork oak seems to allow it to happen, as if it were swaying while its strips of flesh are being pulled off. The color that is uncovered seems to beat, to sing.

A hot earth red.

And then time does its work. Nine years will pass before those hands come back for the newly formed child. Nine summers until the next harvest.

But sometimes wounds are made that never heal. Damage is done to the bark when the cork isn't stripped correctly. When it is wounded, scars are formed on the tree, causing the trunk to no longer be perfectly round. The wound gives way to irregularity, to imperfection, to breakage. To the knot.

And touching a wound that no longer pulses inside that dead cork oak was when my father told me how old it was. The tree that was a stop along the path could very easily be three hundred years old.

Since the publication of my poetry collection *Field Notebook*, stories and details that were never before told or thought important in my home have come to light.

A first book is like a first cell.

My father often gives me ideas, tells me stories that suddenly pop into his head or that he picks up from his friends or from his outings as a veterinarian. That day, next to the tree, the name of a woman I didn't know and had never heard of came up for the first time: my great-great-grandmother Josefa.

The first thing I learned about her was that she loved cork oaks and the land. That my grandmother Teresa referred to her as Grandma Pepa. That she was a strong-willed woman, that she was the one who ran the house and made the decisions. She was the brains and heart of the house. The lifeline, like the aorta, that sustained everyone and kept them alive.

Because Pepa, who was born between 1860 and 1870, didn't only run her house. She prepared meals for everyone, for her own family, for the shepherds, for the day laborers, for those who worked with her day in and day out. They were all one family. She organized the work, prepared for slaughtering, and also took care of all the housework. She was the one who kept track of the finances. Her husband, my great-great-grandfather, was a hard worker, but he didn't have her brains. He walked into the village barefoot, with a mule; he may have been from Extremadura. The first Rodríguez to come to those streets where he would end up settling down. They called him the "*d'avansa*" because he never, ever stopped. But she was the one in charge, which wasn't very common in a mountain village, especially at the time she was born. At nightfall, all her children had to come see her, tell her how their day had gone—making her like someone who reads a story to her children every night to help them fall asleep—so calm would come and she could rest.

They had a small parcel of ground. The little Rodríguez finca. Through hard work, they were able to have a little vegetable garden, a small olive grove, and a piece of land with cork oaks and olive trees. I seem to remember that a river crossed through it. You don't know how important water is until you don't have any. More so in the country.

Her, the head and heart.

Him, the hands.

In the past people didn't have to wait for their parents to die to gain access to the land or property they owned. At a certain age it was no longer possible to work as much. People passed their land on to their children while they were still alive. Maybe it was a way to be certain, a way to hold on. To see how life continues to do its work.

My great-great-grandmother Josefa left a little piece of land to each of her children. But the ritual at nightfall continued to be observed after they were grown. The mother still had to know about each child's work and hands so she could go to sleep peacefully. It's funny how family quirks and traditions are also inherited, even if they take other shapes, and learn how to fit into other masks and developments. My paternal great-grandfather, Juan Sánchez, couldn't go to bed without checking that all the goats had returned safe and sound to the corral from the fields. That all those that had left in the morning had returned. He knew perfectly well, without witnessing the births, which nanny birthed each of the kid goats. This quirk bordered on obsession, and it was so well known throughout the town that a carnival song was composed for him: "'El Pez' has already died / he was buried with his mother, / he gave his soul to God and his goats to Juan Sánchez." I know this story because my father wrote it down. His doctoral dissertation began with this little song, a kind of dedication. Again I think of that invisible narrative, these quirks that are passed down and succeed one another: I came across these verses rummaging through my father's books, looking for stories about animals and trees, photographs, and anecdotes about my family.

The father turns and looks at the daughter. And he tells her that it's not the same tree, but that she could use it to tell a story, to provide the backbone for a book that does not yet exist. And the daughter laughs, because the father, even if he doesn't know it, in his own way, also creates literature.

My great-great-grandmother knew all of her trees extremely well, even though she could no longer go to see them as she had before. Because age, just as it had done with the trees, also did its work on her. She knew perfectly well which oak or cork oak her children were talking about. Because she was still there, with the trees, even if she didn't see them or touch them. That was her genealogy. A room of bark and branches of her own.

The father tells her and allows space for magic. The

daughter wants to retain this in her head. She doesn't want to take her hands off the trunk. She wants to stay there, in that moment that carries the name of a woman and her story out of the shadows. A woman of her family, of her blood. Who might have walked the same path that they've walked on. Who touched the same trees, who rested in the same place.

Ever since the image of the story appeared, the daughter can't get it out of her head. It has become a kind of amulet. Something she likes to carry with her and doesn't want to forget for anything in the world.

When Pepa learned that she had only a few years left to live, and she could no longer walk or take care of herself, she asked to be carried out in a kind of chair to see the oldest and most beautiful cork oak she had. She wanted to say goodbye to her favorite tree.

That summer they stripped its cork. And Pepa sensed, somehow, that neither she nor the tree would live long enough to be there for the next extraction.

Father and daughter decide to continue on. Their steps are waiting for them. Then will come the footprints, a last look at the dead tree still standing, that will be waiting for them on their next visit. But, before they go, they sink their hands into the ground, rummaging through the leaves that the cork oaks replace every year but that never leave the tree completely bare. Between the smell and the moisture, they gather cork oak acorns. Bitter acorns the animals will eat when there's nothing else, when they have no other choice.

They take the acorns out of the leaf litter and put them in their pockets.

When the end of winter approaches and they sense the beginning of spring, they'll take them out again.

They'll plant them far from their point of origin. They'll go to see the seedlings from time to time; they'll place little rocks around them so no one will step on them or harm them, so those who are around them will also be aware of what they cannot see but is underground. So they stop as they pass by, observe, wonder.

They care.

Like the favorite cork oak, like the first cell.

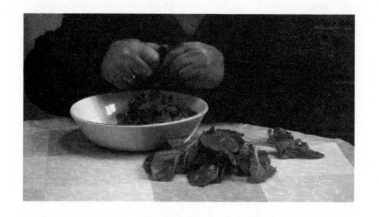

CHAPTER 3

Grandmother: Garden

It's a strange feeling. Walking down the streets of a place where everyone recognizes you. They know where you come from, what you do, where you live. Who you are.

In my town, as in all towns, people who aren't from the place, and don't have any ties to it, are called "outsiders." They stroll through the streets peeking into the open doors, trying to see what lies beyond the vestibules, going into the bars and shops as if they were embarrassed, hesitating, almost unwilling to make any noise. They whisper questions about names they don't know, as if speaking any louder would highlight that they are only passing through, that they don't intend to return. They want to go unnoticed, but visitors here are immediately recognized.

It's a strange feeling. The fact that everyone recognizes you but you feel like an imposter, like a phony outsider. I always say "my town," but I wasn't born there. That place I belong to irremediably: the small mountains that shelter it, that land of hills and trails where all my family comes from, where I always return.

I was born in Córdoba, but I don't have any attachment or ties to the city. I don't feel like a Cordobesa any more than I feel like I am from the town. It's as if I'm in no-man's-land. A wall clock pendulum that goes back and forth but never stops. It doesn't choose and it doesn't remain. The bond is different; I wouldn't mind leaving this city and never coming back. I have an innate, intrinsic, inexplicable need for my town. And not only for its streets but for the entire region it belongs to. The surrounding fields, the streams, the trees, the flocks that make their presence known at dusk. Life happening over and over again without the need for anyone to observe it or point it out.

In my town everyone greets me. Everybody knows me. They say good morning, goodbye; they say, "We're headin' up there again, no?" when they guess the route I'm taking through their streets. I don't know most of them. I might recognize some of their faces, their names, their nick-names. I can sense their ages, their ties to my family. I could guess where their hands and voices are leading them. But I'm always the one who is recognized. Even though I've grown up and stopped playing on their streets. Everyone knows my name. Everyone recognizes my genealogy. They always stop, say hello, ask about my siblings and the rest of my family. Because even though I wasn't born there, I be-long in a certain way to them and their customs.

> "Look, that one belongs to Carmen la gordita, the chubby one."

One of my favorite rural words is *venero*, natural spring, source.

I hold on to the first and third dictionary definitions:

from vein

1: (n) a source of supply; *especially*: a source of water issuing from the ground.

3: (n) origin and beginning of something.

I like to think of myself that way. That I am one of those molecules that rises to the surface at the source of the Huéznar River, in a town near my own, where some of my an-cestors also come from. The beginning. The origin. The start.

The first time I sat next to the spring and looked into the pool of water and its bubbles, I couldn't help but think of the women who came before me, sitting like me, in the same position, resting, or maybe not thinking at all, just watching those first trickles of water being born. And it doesn't just happen to me there, it happens to me everywhere there is water and there is any relationship with my family.

I'm obsessed with shorelines. Because of what the river drags along and what is left on the banks. Stones, mud, twigs. Those inhabitants the water can't handle and leaves on the banks. And even if they don't join the course of the water they let themselves be carried away. They are off-spring of the erosion that shapes them over and over with the force of the water. But I don't like to think this change happens by getting knocked about. I'd rather imagine the force of the water like a mother rocking and soothing her children, transforming them while she too, without realizing it, also changes. And that, despite the moisture and the changing seasons, they are still recognizable.

I didn't know it, but my grandmother Carmen was born and grew up in the country, near a river. When I ask her what her life was like there, how she spent her childhood, she laughs and becomes a child once again. She doesn't want to remember. Despite her hands and the years, she hasn't forgotten the work there and would rather not remember.

She grew up in a little house, with her parents, grandparents, and siblings. Surrounded by chickens and turkeys outside, with no running water or electricity, taking care of the olive trees and the family vegetable garden. From a young age, she had to take food to the men working in the fields every day by herself, an hour's journey by foot. She carried little pots in an *ataero*, as she calls it, a kind of yoke, whether it was hot or cold. Sometimes, along the way, she'd reach inside a pot and eat a little bit without anyone noticing.

They made their own bread at home and she helped my great-grandmother knead it in the kneading trough. When I was told the location of the mill where they took the wheat I had to go. I needed to follow the same path they did. Imagine that weight they carried on my own body. Get my feet wet, think about espadrilles. I put my hands in the gap where the door should be. I knocked on the air a few times, let them, the ghosts, pass in front of me, talk to the miller, no bargaining or special treatment, and then, as they left, the father's hand resting on the daughter's shoulder. And with support, conforming, without complaint, in a whisper: "The miller always keeps what he wants."

I think again of the strangeness, of the sensation of walking over a piece of land again and again without knowing that on that ground there was once a small garden, a little corral nearby with a goat for my grandmother to milk and bottle-feed her sister Lola every day, because my great-grandmother had no breast milk. Picking up those meaningless stones, scattered and covered with moss where once there was a house that sheltered an entire family, barely lit by the light of an oil lamp. Looking for the fruit trees that were used as a boundary, imagining them, raising your hands in the air, like someone picking fruit and leaving it in the basket, making a movement to remember, to recognize yourself there.

The source, the spring is still there. She has turned into a sister of time, and of all of us who have gone there. Sometimes I think of her as defiant; she's the only one still standing. She shelters a few fig trees and a quince tree abandoned to a state of neglect. There are also lilacs. My grandmother's brother would always go there and bring a sprig back home. Water, again, like a survivor, like a reproach for all of us who left and didn't want to return.

≈

I travel by myself a lot. I often go days sleeping away from home. I eat in bars and cafes, always alone. And I become that stranger who interrupts the course of the days in the towns I pass through for work. Most of these places are filled with men who turn and look at me when I walk in. A few break the silence and ask me about my work, the reason for my visit, if the truck parked outside the door is mine. This last question I find especially funny, and, whenever I answer, they always look at me in surprise: I have never been afraid. Because I haven't been aware of any fear myself until my interns, who sometimes join me in my fieldwork, have asked me about being afraid, about spending so much time alone on the road, in unfamiliar places, in places full of men.

Until recently I thought I was like those women. It might be that I'm getting older, because these past few years I see them younger and I can't help but feel a protective instinct. I don't want them to get hurt. And this is something I not only think about with my students, but also with my family and friends. The vulnerability of those I love, a new feeling that has burst into my home like someone sitting at the table waiting to be fed.

I couldn't help but ask my grandmother if she ever felt afraid when she was living in the country, when she went to work alone day after day, when she was left alone because her children left and my grandfather died. Alone with her garden and her chickens. When she is still alone and doesn't want to call the doctor to come see her. My grandmother replies:

"If I have food I'm not afraid of anything."

Only once did I see something resembling fear on her face. Although it was more like a kind of distrust. One day, peeking into her room from the doorway, I saw a flash. It was the image of the Virgin she has on her bedside table. It had gold threads on it. I'm not religious, but before I realized it I was holding the Virgin in my hands, pressed against my chest. Half angry, my grandmother told me not to show it "around too much." No one should know she had it. The little holy image is more than two hundred years old, from when the town was just a small village. My grandmother Carmen doesn't know where her grandmother got it from. But she has kept it ever since and it's who she looks at before she goes to sleep.

She doesn't want to take it out of her house or show it

to anyone in church because "those sanctimonious women will take it away" from her.

We all need something to hold on to. A place to belong to, something to be part of. I cling to my grandmother Carmen's little vegetable garden. With its green gate and its thick, quicklime walls. When you turn down her street, you can see it from above. My book *Field Notebook* was born there one morning when I was helping my mother pick laurel while, along the fence across the street, the neighbor's sheep began to call their lambs. I remember that I felt the need to look at the ground, at the soil, where there were always potatoes, and to dig my hands down and get them dirty, looking for roots that are no longer there. The neighbor in the house next door started playing fandangos. One of those moments when everything seems to make sense.

My grandmother doesn't know how to write. She went to a school for the illiterate for a few days, but she had to leave because she had to work with her family in the countryside. She worked a lot, more than some of the men in her family. Today she laughs remembering her maternal grandfather. In the village they called him Paciencia, patience, because he'd start rigging his mule at seven in the morning and by ten o'clock he still hadn't finished.

She has spent much of her life alone. Even before her husband died. For years my grandfather José would spend eight or nine months out of the year working in Switzerland. He returned to the village for the remaining months to work in the olive harvest and in the cooperative. They didn't call each other. He sent his family postcards, letters, photographs. There's a photo of him that's like a little heartbeat. My grandfather appears in his foreign room, smiling at the camara, turning his eyes to the task, packing his suitcase to return home. The image is blurry, but despite the years and the haze on the paper, it says so much. My grandmother and her young children received his letters, and it was my mother or their neighbor Rosario who wrote the replies to my grandfather.

My grandmother doesn't know how to write, but she takes care of the garden by herself. She gathers the seeds, dries them, stores them in small jars in the pantry. Germinates them when the time is right. She knows how to care for the chickens, prepare the olives, make preserves, set the potatoes on a piece of cardboard in the loft. She knows how to prepare a vegetable garden for the cold, whitewash the walls of her house. Go to the cooperative and its olive trees, keep track of the house expenses. She's a strong woman, and she's never been bothered by being alone. When I started living by myself she prepared an "independent woman's" trousseau for me, with cups, teapots, plates, and coffee pots. She gave me my great-grandmother Rosario's coffee set so I could have the items on display at home, so I could be proud of them.

> "I'll prepare the trousseau and give it to you, but you don't have to get married, you'll manage just fine on your own."

I like to open the small storage room off her patio and touch the scale painted in blue, a little chipped, resting on a table covered with a plastic oilcloth filled with holes. My brother José and I loved to play with it. We'd imitate my grandmother when she'd sell eggs and vegetables from the garden to her neighbors. She never let her children play with it. The scale, which belonged to her mother Rosario, is now more than a hundred years old. It has a knowledge of hands and stories we'll never understand. Now the room is always closed. Surrounded by wicker baskets and empty glass jars, the scale is there alone, holding a few small potatoes, a box of matches, and a sprig of fennel tied with a scrap of cloth, to season the olives.

My grandmother's hands know nothing of books and notebooks, but they do know about the cold and soil.

My grandmother Carmen laughs again when I ask her why we're called *las gorditas*, the chubby ones. Carmen la gordita. Her second name, by which everyone knows her, she inherited from her grandmother Dolores. She was a big baby, born chubby. In times of hunger and scarcity, that was a sign of health and happiness. And from Dolores to this day.

I've also inherited the name.

I'm also part of that lineage of women of the land, with their hands full of corn to feed their chickens, with their hands in the hands of those who caught the hares, who know about quicklime and the places where poachers hide, who rise up, in spite of everything, like the knees of all women, pocked with dirt and little stones from picking up and collecting olives. That tree of women that could be an olive tree, a fig tree, a laurel, a rose bush, a patio filled with flowerpots, a sprig of mint and parsley, a lemon tree, some tomato plants, a flower bed bursting with blossoms.

I am also part of Carmen la gordita, with her generous thighs, without the waist of a wasp she had when she married, with her hands under the table skirt, looking for the heat of a *brasero de picón* while she goes on chopping chard and talking about the weather and the town's entanglements.

Part of Carmen la gordita, the one who was the first to go down to the garden to water it in the summer, alone, while her husband was working construction in a cold and distant country, who was inseparable from her sister-in-law Antonia, who was like a sister to her, who had a beautiful courtyard and never stopped asking all the other women in the town for pot cuttings.

I'm also part of la gordita, a woman who has never seen the sea and who isn't worried about dying without seeing it. She prefers to remember swimming along the riverbank, always with her door open for her neighbors, sitting outside every cool summer night on the only bench on the street, pulling out as many chairs as necessary so that everyone could have their place. All these women alone with their children, contemplating the stars, taking care of each other.

Carmen can no longer walk. Now it's my mother and I who go down to the garden. The ones who imitate the ceremonies of their trees with their hands. The ones who go back inside happy to tell her about her vegetables. The ones who prepare a nice bouquet of roses to accompany her in the living room. The ones who never stop asking about seeds, recipes, names, stories, places.

Every time I come back my grandmother Carmen is sitting in the kitchen, waiting for me. Depending on the season, she's prepared a dish with figs or pomegranates. She always has, ever since I was a little girl. These fruits carry my grandmother's scent, her name, her origin. Because the branches that continue to grow in the orchard are daughters of the trees her great-grandfather planted in the field where she grew up as a child. And she, when she married, brought the seeds to the town grove so they could give shelter and food to the rest of us. Like the natural spring, reminding us again and again of the origin, the root, the beginning. Like the seeds that are always kept, as a rite, as a way to remember over and over where we came from and where we should go.

Maybe I want to recognize myself that way too:

To belong to the clan of women who wear a spike of grain

stuck to their chest. Far from the sea. To care with hands covered with dirt, pulling up weeds. To season the olives, prepare the preserves in a bain-marie.

To set the basket with the eggs and vegetables on the ground, to close the gate with both hands, and stand up like my grandmother when she used to go down to the garden herself. She would stand and smile, as if saying goodbye to the place, breathing a sigh, making life stand still while I watched her pull up her stockings and grab the basket again as if it were nothing.

To want, to cling to.

Clinging again and again to that genealogy with the voice and memory of a pantry full of little jars of seeds, spices, and seasonings, of weights and baskets that never had any qualms about being filled and shared with their loved ones.

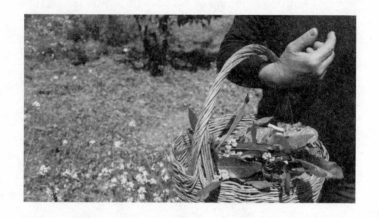

CHAPTER 4

Mamá: Olive Tree

The closest thing to writing I found in college was becoming a student intern in the Department of Anatomy and Topographical Neuroanatomy. Dissecting, separating muscles, cleaning arteries and veins, learning how to poke around without damaging the tissue. Filling the circulatory and lymphatic systems with dyes, being careful not to break any bones, not to damage the skin or hair of the animals I worked with. My hands always wet, the smell of formaldehyde pulsing in my lungs and on my fingers.

Learning to dissect and plastinate became a private room of my own. A refuge where I could go between classes, a place where, even if I was alone, I felt accompanied. I didn't feel judged or under anyone's watchful eye.

It's difficult to be the daughter and granddaughter of. The expectations your parents place on you, as a rule, are quite high. I studied veterinary medicine in the same city as my grandfather and my father. I was already starting on a steep incline. My father is a professor at the university, and, although I was never his student, I had to carry that around with me. Neither of us wanted to be associated with the other for any reason at all.

My classmates laughed, though not maliciously, when they saw me taking out collections of poems and novels on breaks between classes. One professor asked me how it was that I had time to read with all that I had to study. I was still the weirdo I had always felt like I was.

During those years, my relationship with my father worsened. I went from being the apple of his eye to a brooding teenager who was never good enough. I went from being the kid who, from the age of three, wanted to be a woman veterinarian to a troubled girl who was totally disappointed with her career choice. For my father, the poems I'd write here and there on the sly between my notes were signs that I had my head in the clouds. I had to dedicate myself to my

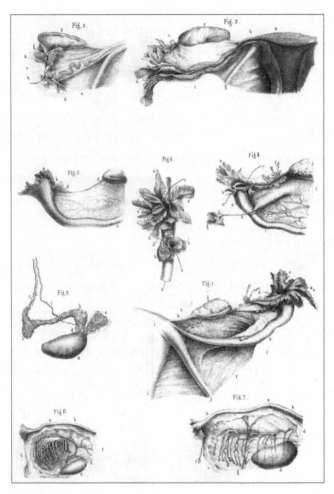

Uterine tubes and ovaries by Bourgery

studies, to earning my degree; I had to focus. Everything else was a waste of time.

Veterinary medicine is a long-distance race. It requires discipline, sacrifice, and time, a lot of time. I was frustrated that I couldn't have time for literature and writing. I hated that hackneyed and so-often-repeated phrase "I'm a science person" that some of my classmates would say to me when they saw me in the library studying, surrounded by novels and books of poetry. It's also true that the educational system has made sure that we learn this little song by heart.

That's why the dissecting room became the calm and solitude I needed. I didn't write but I used my hands. I could sample, attempt, make mistakes, without anyone reprimanding me. I wasn't disappointing anyone. I wasn't pursuing any particular end. To complete the preparation, to exhibit what the one who dissects and prepares the body wants shown, to turn the animal into an object of contemplation. Into a beautiful enticement that does not hide, where all eyes look.

Although it may not seem like it, dissection and writing share many things. Patience is one of them. Both with words and with the scalpel, through trial and error, you end up finding something that convinces you. Sometimes it doesn't have a name, but you sense that it's there, that you're on the right track. A heartbeat you hear that becomes an impulse you follow.

My anatomy professor introduced me to Bourgery and his treatises full of illustrations. Looking for information about him, I found an observation by the Savoyard philosopher Joseph de Maistre in one of my professor's notes:

> All science begins with a mystery…An idea that seems so clear to us is nothing more than a glimmer between two abysses.

A mystery, a light surrounded by darkness. What Maistre promulgated could be fully extrapolated as a hand that begins to write.

The hands, before finding the word, intuit, palpate, recognize. They are blind until they find that light that ends up becoming writing. And in this search, they find other hands that provide shelter and companionship. And it is during times of greater darkness that other hands are most necessary, when the light they give off guides more than ever before.

My mother has been a complete stranger to me for years.

I didn't want to look like her; I didn't want to end up like her. My teenage self didn't understand how my mother had become a perfect housewife, in my father's shadow, always there for and with us. I was often angry at her. Always cooking, cleaning, never resting. She got on my nerves because I thought she didn't have any concerns, that she owed everything to my father, that she didn't aspire to anything. Today I am aware that it's unfair and wrong but I need to write it down because at the time I thought that's how it was. And I think something like this has happened to many daughters with our mothers. That's why feminism has been so important to so many women of my generation. Because it has become those determined, unshakable hands that have fearlessly taken off the blindfold we had on our eyes and taught us to look beyond, to change our point of view, to tear down the foundations and the truths we held as absolutes.

My mother has been that glimmer in the darkness. Not only for me, but also for my brothers and my father. I think a lot about when we were children and about my mother alone, in a city that wasn't hers, without family, while my father worked in South America for long periods of time. Now that we are talking about equality and conciliation. Now that I have become one of many hands raised up and part of a generation that makes demands. Now I think about her. About everything she did for us. And what she couldn't do.

My mother's name is Carmen, like her mother. Since she was a child she had to help her parents and grandparents in the olive grove. Sometimes she would run away to play in the stream, do something mischievous and hide so she wouldn't have to return to the olive harvest. Once, my grandmother told me that my mother disappeared for so long that my great-grandfather, followed by the donkey, called for her crying among the olive trees. He shouted between his wailing: "Carmelina, Carmelina, where have you gone?"

My mother's favorite thing to do was to take a basket, curl up inside it, and roll down the hill into a shady spot below. Nothing ever happened to her because my great-grandfather Sastre arrived in time to stop the naughty girl from falling into the water.

There are moments in our lives that just happen but they stay with us forever. My mother always remembers her grandfather tiptoeing on top of his mule so he could reach the highest branches and knock the olives down with a stick. She guided the animal while my great-grandfather became a tightrope walker among the olive trees. Maybe she learned the trade, the profession, without knowing it. She was already giving a glimpse of that hand that shelters and guides her loved ones.

When I ask my mother about her early years, there's never a clear separation between play and work. "Playing," she helped pick olives or pile up twigs to prepare the *cisco*, or charcoal, that would later rest in the *braseros de picón* that would heat her house. "Playing," she helped her mother clean the house, cook, and take care of the garden and the chickens. She tells me that she only had one doll, which she played at being a mother with, that she washed the few clothes it had and sometimes put curlers made from paper balls in her hair. She and her friends would use cardboard boxes and some weeds from the field and little stones and they'd play store: one would sell and another would buy what she needed for cooking. They recreated what they saw at home, preparing themselves, playfully, for what awaited most of them in the future. The Three Kings didn't bring gifts, but what was really needed in a humble village house in the 1960s: socks, coats, blankets, a dress. Basically, clothing.

Out of that childhood of games that replicated an unequal system for women, my mother moved on to an adolescence dedicated to work. Because she was the one, being *la hermana de un hermano único*, the daughter in a family with only one son, who had to leave school at the age of fourteen to go to work in the olive harvest. She didn't quit, she didn't speak out, she didn't complain. That's how it was. Everything for her brother, nothing for her. While he went to school every day, my mother had to walk for an hour to the family olive grove. Her father went out earlier, she and her mother, only once they'd cleaned the house and prepared the food to take for the day's work, which they'd cooked the night before. My mother insists: your grandfather always prepared the *café con migas* and in the olive grove he was the one who heated the pot over the fire and called to us by raising his voice among the olive trees with "familia, come, come and eat."

An exercise I do now is compare what my mother and I have done in our lives at different ages. While she was a housewife in miniature and worked in the fields, my brother and I went to school without a care in the world, with a table full of food waiting for us when we returned. While I could decide what to study, what to do in the future, my mother was still on her knees, picking up olives in the cold and rain, drawing water from the well and bringing it to her family.

I think about my father, too. In his professional career. And I know that neither he nor any of his children would have come to anything if it hadn't been for my mother. There's nothing to celebrate. She was denied independence, education, and the ability to make her own decisions. My mother's story is the same as that of so many women in this country who dedicated their entire lives to their families, putting themselves last. They never got sick, they never complained, there was never a problem. These weren't extraordinary qualities or powers granted by the grace of God. Only that they had to live in an era of machismo in which women were reduced to the domestic space, where they became mothers and companions. Where their voice wasn't as loud and the walls became boundaries they couldn't cross. And, of course, this is not something exclusive to our towns, this inequality reached the majority of women in our territory, while their male siblings were the chosen ones, the ones who enjoyed their freedom and an education. Everything for the male; *todas*…all women, *hermanas de un hijo único*…sisters of an only child.

Machismo didn't only reach women like my mother. My father always speaks to me with great affection about his great-aunts, Amelia and Ana, who studied commerce and were among the first women to work at the Central Bank of Spain. They lived in Seville. And they remained unmarried. They were no longer from the town, but they didn't fit in in the city either. They were two independent women who, although they had each other, had been forced to be alone; they chose to educate themselves and to work. They had been left in no-man's-land.

There's a portrait in my maternal grandparents' house that I need to look at every time I go back to their town. When I was little, I thought it was a picture of my mother. Until one time I said to her: "You look so pretty in that picture, Mamá."

But the girl in the photo was never my mother. It was her cousin Candidita. She emigrated, like most of my maternal family, to towns and suburbs in Catalonia. There they would begin other lives, other jobs. As waitresses, housekeepers, guards, maids, service ladies. A distant family cousin was one of the first female cab drivers there. They would come in the summer and open up their houses, as if they'd never left, and continue their life in the town as if nothing had happened. They always went back with their suitcases and baskets full of black pudding and vegetables from the town. There, women continued to repeat the customs of the place where they came from. Songs, recipes, habits. They sent letters until the telephone arrived. They continued to take their chairs out into the fresh air, into the streets, gathering and taking care of each other, as if their town were not a place but a small animal that each carried inside and that asked to be cared for and fed every day.

My aunt Candida looked identical to my mother. They were the same age. She died of meningitis when she was eighteen. She came back from high school with a headache that never went away and was taken to a hospital far from home. I only met her through her mother who, as soon as she returned to town on the first day of summer, came to see my mother and touch her face and hug her, to be close, in a way, to the daughter she had lost.

While her cousin Candida went to high school, my mother started working in a sewing workshop. My grandmother wanted her to learn a trade at least. So her hands would know more than cold and dirt. She worked twelve-hour shifts in the workshop. They paid her very little. And on the days she didn't go to the workshop she had to continue helping the family in the olive harvest and in the garden. On her day off she helped my grandmother with the housework. She always tells me: When she was fifteen she had to wash and iron her own clothes. After washing and ironing everyone else's.

For my mother, meeting my father had to be a kind of liberation. Although she moved from her father's house to her husband's, leaving her town and settling in Córdoba was good for her. She could decide not to be accountable to so many people. To start a life where she made her own small decisions and created a home for her children.

I used to get angry when my mother said that she didn't like the country, that she didn't feel like going back to her town. That she didn't want to go live there. Now I understand, how is she going to like it if for her it meant work and sacrifice?

For her, the countryside is not a place for contemplation or for rest. It means cold, rain, wounded hands, and no power over her own life. It means being in the shadow of her father and her grandfather. Obeying, serving, giving. Always being attentive to others. Caring for them. Never looking out for herself. Always becoming the last one.

My mother's relationship (and that of so many women) with the rural environment becomes an extra-terrestrial story when compared to the relationship so many men have with it. I think of Miguel Delibes and Félix Rodríguez de la

Fuente. How different the countryside can be depending on your gender, your family, and the circumstances you were born into. While some contemplated, observed, cared for, hunted in, and, in the end, enjoyed the countryside, others worked tirelessly in it and for others.

It is obvious why there are no women writers from my mother's generation in this country who write from and about rural areas. Thanks to feminism, we have recovered and know about the women who were part of the Generation of '27. We know that they existed, that they had a voice, and that they wrote. That they were strong, independent, and talented. The same is not true for women in our rural community. Rural women couldn't tell their stories because most of them couldn't write. Because they were denied the pleasure of reading, going to school, being able to decide what to do, what training they wanted. They were denied culture altogether. Before them lay only the countryside they worked in. Just a house with four walls where they cleaned, cooked, and cared for others. Even they think they have nothing interesting to say. That their life is a conse-quence of their home and family, that this is their place. So where do they find recognition? Because, as Berger wrote, "every culture acts in general as a mirror that allows the subject to recognize himself, or, at least to recognize those parts of himself that are socially acceptable. Those who suffer from cultural deficiencies have fewer opportunities to recognize themselves."

My grandmother and mother don't want to write. They think their lives and their stories have no value. That's why I write. They have a voice; I want to serve as a weaver, that *altavoz* and platform. I want them and so many other rural women to recognize themselves and recover their space. So they can build their home, so they can tell their stories without fear or shame. Without feeling less than, inferior to anyone else.

This fall my mother, while we were with my grandmother sitting around the *brasero* shelling beans, began to talk out of the blue about the swing her father made for her in an oak tree by the little house in the olive grove. She was smiling. I kept thinking of her as a little girl, swinging, gaining momentum, smiling.

That afternoon we decided to go there, to see the oak tree that cradled my mother, to walk the path she had walked to the olive grove so many times. I admit that for me it was an adventure. My mother hardly ever talks to me about her childhood. My mother's life before she was my mother was a mystery to me. We left the village, walking for quite a while, stepping in the footsteps of my child-mother and so many ancestors who had walked the same path accompanied by their animals to the olive-laden branches. She kept telling me things she had never told me before. As if this return to childhood had activated something in her, as if this path she'd walked so many times before had become something new and unknown.

But we had to turn back. They had fenced off part of the path. And the gates were padlocked. Although we had the right to pass because it was a drovers' path, and therefore a public lane, we turned around. The oak tree and the invisible swing remained only in our memory. We also left behind the tracks of so many animals, shepherds, and laborers that were still there, invisible despite the passage of time, like a mark that weighs on all those who knew that *cañada*, that ravine which is also a drovers' path, was a path for everyone. A *sendero* or trail that was shared with the flocks and the hands that guided them. We went back, but it seemed that it was the hundred-year-old olive trees with their hollows and the sounds and smells of the countryside that were leaving.

Entering town, my mother remembered that she needed laurel. She put on her mother's boots. She tied her hair back. She took the keys to the garden's green gate. She grabbed a basket that held only a pair of scissors and the remains of some dry leaves. I sat there, looking at her. She sang as she cut the sprigs. Carefully, she was putting them in the wicker basket without dropping any leaves. That day she told me there were women who knew how to read the future with leaves from the laurel tree. I, a little hypnotized by the increasingly strong smell, couldn't take my eyes off the tree's flowers. Some of them fell off when she picked up the sprigs. They reminded me of something, but I didn't know what.

Later that afternoon, going down to the orchard again but this time alone—this time it was me wearing my grandmother's boots and carrying my own basket—I remembered. The flowers reminded me of that treatise on anatomical illustrations by Bourgery. That book that had accompanied me in the dissection room. Only the flowers that appeared in the atlas were pink and weren't part of any tree. The flowers that had no place in that orchard and existed only in my head weren't flowers at all. They were the lateral extremities of the uterine tubes. Their infundibula. One of my favorite parts in dissection of the female reproductive tract.

The nest.

The shelter.

The source.

The lullaby.

A glimmer between two abysses.

NOTE ON THE COVER

When a baby is born in a Navajo Nation community, the parents cut the umbilical cord and bury it in their sheep pen. In this way the bond between the newest inhabitant of the tribe with the animals and with their land is created and materialized.

"We were created with our sheep," says one of the songs sung in a Navajo ceremony. For them, their relationship with livestock and pastoralism is so important that it is even reflected in the origin and creation story of the tribe:

Changing Woman (celestial being) gave birth to the sheep and the goats. She soaked the earth with the amniotic fluid from her placenta, which enveloped the ruminants. And so from the ground germinated and sprouted the plants that would feed their animals, which they would then care for and take across the land. Such is the command for the Navajo people.

From that amniotic fluid and that first woman's placenta, pastoralism, extensive livestock production, and shepherds were born. This utterly unique and important union of territory, animal, and person.

Since I was a child, I've been fascinated by all the stories, tales, lullabies, and ceremonies of indigenous communities. Maybe because most are filled with animals, trees, and territory. With people who care for and celebrate the environment they live in. With grandparents who tell stories to their grandchildren so that this bond between the animal and the territory endures. With parents who continue to believe in making possible that union between their children and the land they inhabit and that feeds them.

I wasn't raised in an indigenous community, but I grew up surrounded by animals. My family let me fall down and cover my knees with mud and cuts. They taught me how to whistle and run after the herd of goats we had, to learn to push the rock roses aside with my hands, to drink from the stream with a cork dipper, to follow after the chickens with a basket to collect their eggs, to pick vegetables in the garden and fruit from the trees my grandfather planted for every grandchild who was born. To stack the firewood, to bind the top-graft cuttings in scraps of cloth, to make queso fresco in the afternoons with the milk all the village goat-herders brought the night before.

My family taught me to care for everything around me, to help my grandparents and to never get tired of listening to them.

That is why Joaquim Gomis Serdañons's photograph is on the cover. His daughter Odette hugs a baby goat in the French region of Megève, in 1939, during the Gomis family's exile.

For me, this is the sibling bond of the Navajo baby's umbilical cord to the land where the animals, which are part of the family, rest. That bond with the rural environment and its inhabitants I have had since I was a child, the strong relationship that has made it possible for me to always be in my day-to-day life and that, at the end of the day, has influenced me as much in my personal life as my professional.

To some it might seem that this photograph idealizes or remains on the surface of the rural environment. They're mistaken. Those of us who love and defend the rural environment and everything that inhabits it (seeds, native breeds, trees, territory, towns, biodiversity, and ultimately, culture and heritage), do so because of that strong bond that has grown in us since we were children. Because our families and our communities were part of, cared for, gave importance to, grafted that bond onto our childhood. That's why this photograph is so important to me. The little I know for certain in this life is that if I hadn't had the childhood I had, I wouldn't be a field veterinarian or a writer today. This book wouldn't exist; it wouldn't be in your hands.

Every day it becomes clearer to me why I write: for them. For that seed, like that umbilical cord buried in the ground, that continues to sprout in my day-to-day life.

My link to the land and the animals, my roots, my place in the tribe.

I also intend for Gomis's photograph to be a reflection for all those who are fathers and mothers, for those who want to be, and for those who don't.

Our rural community will die if we don't know how to transmit its importance and care to those who come after us. And not only our rural community but all the biodiversity that lives in it, our towns, our customs, our stories. Our culture, like that, without the adjective *rural*, because it is culture, and it belongs to everyone. We must learn to look and transmit. Ask our grandmothers, our mothers. Give importance to our history and to our villages. Ask, tell, listen, question ourselves, again and again. Look beyond. Get our hands dirty. Let those who are to come, the children of the future, get dirty as well. Soak up the land and animals, the stories of their elders, shake hands with them; let them want to visit and inhabit a house filled with roots and heritage that has yet to be built.

Create a bond and nurture it.

This is the only way that our rural environment will not disappear and will continue to exist.

We were here, one day we were alive here.

GLOSSARY

Introduction: An Invisible Narrative

altavoz (altavoces): Sound system, like a speaker, but also a speaker, like a spokesperson to speak for those who have been silenced.

field veterinarian: Not just a veterinarian who works in the country, but one who travels distances following livestock herds, conducting research and working with pastoralists from different regions and with diverse livestock.

livestock producers: From the Spanish word *ganadero*, though *ganadera*—the feminine gender of the noun—is most often used in the original Spanish-language edition of this book; in other contexts it could be translated as ranchers, cattlewomen, or cattlemen.

Medio Rural: This Spanish term appears in English translation throughout the book. It can be translated in multiple ways depending on context; some of its uses in this book include "rural environment," "rural community," "rural areas," and "rural towns."

transhumant: Adjective form of *transhumance*, a form of pastoralism or nomadism organized around the migration of livestock between mountain pastures in warm seasons and lower altitudes of valleys during the winter months. Could also be translated as nomadic, migratory, migrating, on the move to new pastures.

1. A Genealogy of the Countryside

destello (destellos): A flash, a glimmer, glint, sparkle, flare, gleaming.

ellas: Them, feminine.

extensive livestock production: From the Spanish term *ganadería extensiva*, livestock production that allows for a more natural existence for the animals and is more respectful of the land; the opposite of intensive livestock production, in which animals are raised in confinement buildings or in massive feedlots.

2. A Feminism of Sisters and Land

Bologna Plan: Or the Bologna Process, the harmonization of standards for higher education across almost fifty countries in Europe, adopted in 1999.

March 8, 2018: March 8 is International Women's Day, also known as 8M in Spain. March 8, 2018, saw an unprecedented mobilization for women's rights in Spain, with millions of

women going on strike to advocate for gender equality in
wages and rights.

territory *(territorio)*: Translated in some places in this book as
"land," this refers to the different regions around Spain, or
even the whole country.

3. The Caring Hand

Catalunya Ramaderes: A collective of women practicing pastoralism, fighting machismo, and promoting animal welfare in
the Catalan countryside. Catalonia (*Catalunya* in the Catalan
language) is an autonomous community in the northeastern
corner of Spain at the foot of the Pyrenees; it consists of four
provinces: Barcelona, Girona, Lleida, and Tarragona.

Ganaderas en Red, or the Women's Ranchers Network: Group
dedicated to challenging the historical status quo of wom-
en's labor going unacknowledged, despite being crucial to
the operations of the farm, by demanding recognition and
decision-making power. "Women of land, wind, and cattle:
the land in the soul, the wind in the hair, and the cattle in the
heart" is their motto.

story of Kalima: Müller and Prandi's article "Rape in the Fields,"
about the abuses against women fieldworkers in Spain, Italy,
and Morocco, was published by *Correctiv*, an online German investigative journalism resource, in April 2018. Lowell
Berman's documentary of the same name, about immigrant
farmworkers in the United States, aired on PBS's *Frontline* in
June 2013.

They don't want it to rain coffee in the fields *(No quieren que llueva
café en el campo)*: From a popular song by Juan Luis Guerra, referring to something extraordinary but unnatural.

5. For a Living Rural Community

lengua: Tongue, as in language spoken, but also the muscular
   organ in the mouth.

2. Great-Great-Grandmother: Cork Oak

bornizo: The cork obtained in the first harvest, which takes place
   when the tree is thirty to fifty years old. From then on, cork
   can be harvested every nine to fourteen years. It is harvested
   entirely by hand; the thick bark is stripped from the trunks,
   essentially skinning the tree of its protective outermost layer.
   Cork trees typically live between 150 and 250 years.

3. Grandmother: Garden

Carmen *la gordita*, the chubby one: A kind of nickname, not in-
   tended to be offensive, but as a term of endearment.

4. Mamá: Olive Tree

café con migas: A dish prepared with leftover, crusty bread. In
   Andalusia it might include sausage; in other places, and most
   likely in this context, it is made with bread, oil, garlic, and bell
   pepper.
Generation of '27: This refers to an influential group of Spanish poets associated with avant-garde art and poetry, including well-known figures like Federico García Lorca, Salvador
   Dalí, and Luis Buñuel. Women members of this group, such
   as María Zambrano, Rosa Chacel, and Maruja Mallo, have received less attention.

NOTE FROM THE TRANSLATOR

Curtis Bauer

I first encountered María Sánchez's books in spring 2019 when I was living in Seville, Spain, though I didn't intend to translate any of them. I read *Field Notebook*, Sánchez's first collection of poems, and then, after reading a review of *Land of Women* in *Babelia*, the literary supplement to the Spanish newspaper *El País*, I bought that book and started reading it on my trip back to the United States to attend a writers conference in Portland, Oregon. Although I had read only half of *Land of Women*, I couldn't stop telling friends and editors at the conference book fair about the memoir, its unique approach to universal issues of ecology, feminism, gender and linguistic equality, and the rural community in Spain, which I had very little trouble linking to the rural community where I grew up. As someone who was born and raised on a small farm in the Midwest, I immediately found parallels between Sánchez's discussion of the "rural problem" (including the silenced voices of women farmers, the dangers of mass grain and livestock production, the perceived lack of culture in rural communities, and the towns and counties emptied of their youth who no longer saw a future connected to the land, agriculture, and livestock raising) in Spain and similar issues in the United States.

One of the strengths rural communities can offer us in times of crisis, Sánchez points out, is that they can be a model for how we live in urban settings. In numerous interviews and lectures she notes how fortunate she has felt to have such a relationship, such a union, such a closeness to the countryside, because she was taught to value it at a young age. But how many children see birds in the cities and don't know their names, or the same with trees, which we rarely know how to identify? One of our urban problems is that we don't know where food comes from or how it is produced. Many children believe milk comes from a factory, not from a cow. *Land of Women* discusses how we can look to the margins, the rural communities, to relearn how to value the natural world. From the urban perspective it is difficult to understand that mass production of twenty thousand cattle removes any connection with the land when only two people work with them; any relationship between animals and people is broken. And, of course, we must not forget that the people who live in the rural communities are citizens like the people who live in cities. We must be rid of the idea that those who live in the country are second-class citizens; they have the same rights to minimum and basic services such as education, health, roads, schools, leisure, and culture.

And yet there's more here that needs consideration in this work, in this translation. You will see numerous words that are no longer so common in our everyday idiom, words you might have to look up, not because they are in Spanish—there are a few of those, but they've mostly settled into our American idiom—but because they have fallen out of use or are not used outside of rural communities. When María Sánchez realized there was a language she grew up with that she didn't have complete access to, she began to be proactive: for her words are like seeds. Part of her work is to collect and sow language, like the seeds stuck to the loins of transhumant animals. I've tried to carry this over in my translation—using language, vocabulary, that is not simplified or necessarily easy, but that urges readers not just to look for the meaning of these terms but to ask their communities about them, to investigate, to create a conversation. Create new conversations that will be fertile ground for talking about our past, our heritage, about the population that inhabits the margins—everywhere that isn't an urban center—and that will urge us to find parallel language that might encourage readers to search for their connection to the land.

In my first meeting with Sánchez I was struck by her engagement with multiple communities: feminist groups, agriculturalists—I use this term to include livestock raisers, pastoralists, farmers, ranchers, veterinarians, anyone connected to the vast field of agriculture—social justice groups, cultural and educational organizations. So who is this book written for; who is the audience? Initially it was for those living in rural areas who have been silenced or forgotten, whose story has never been told. But the reception by urban readers has been surprising: this book has functioned as a catalyst for many readers to look at their family history, and to think about where they come from, who their grandparents were and what they did before they moved to the cities. Do we know the stories of those who came before us? Have we listened to our predecessors, asked them? This book urges us to do that.

We have learned much from the pandemic of 2020, in particular about what, who, we can so easily lose. This is a time for us to reevaluate our roots and look for ways to identify and solidify connections to others. The pandemic has left many of our communities, in particular those in rural areas across the nation, to fend for themselves, something that has often happened before. What is visible is the urban, and the rural is invisible not only in Spain, as Sánchez shows us, but also in the United States. How can we bring attention to the rural communities and rural culture that has so long been overlooked, silenced, forgotten? Included here are the women in these rural communities, those women who are always behind the man, the wife of, the daughter of, the sister of...Accordingly, this translation attempts to address the attention the author gives to gender by amplifying those gender-specific words that are often easily glossed over into gender-neutral English terms, such as in this example in part 1's chapter 5, "For a Living Rural Community":

I'm a simple field veterinarian who is a woman and works in the rural evironment every day. I'm not a woman expert on depopulation, I'm not a woman sociologist, I'm not a woman politician, I'm not a woman specialist, I'm not a woman livestock producer, I'm not a woman farmer, I'm not a woman shepherd, I'm not a woman researcher, I am not.

The import of this project lies in this author's activism. Sánchez is a writer whose life is linked to the land. In one interview she gave about the relationship between her literary work and her work as a field veterinarian, she said that her childhood "cannot be understood without the rural environment, and without the countryside and its animals." During her childhood she spent the weekends surrounded by the family goat and sheep herds and running around the family cheese factory. Her classmates in the city did not understand her universe; therefore, she took refuge in books, discovering García Lorca's *Blood Wedding* and *Yerma*, but she says that her father used to take those books away from her because he considered them inappropriate for an eight-year-old girl.

As the daughter and granddaughter of veterinarians, she

is the first woman in her family to practice a profession traditionally performed by men. She graduated from the University of Córdoba with a degree in veterinary medicine and combined her studies with books of literature and poetry. "When my grandfather passed away," she notes, "I discovered one of his books on veterinary biochemistry from the year 1942, each chapter of which began with a quote from literature. Why can't I be a scientist and dedicate myself to the arts?"

Now, in her early thirties, Sánchez has three publications that have given her recognition throughout the Spanish-speaking world. They are books in which she defends the role of rural women in order to make them visible. Her most recent book, *Almáciga* (*Nursery* or *Greenhouse*), takes her activism a step further. The book is the continuation of her observations in *Land of Women* and contains extensive research on the words of the rural communities around Spain: "The countryside and our rural environments have a unique way of speaking that brings together territory, people, and animals," Sánchez says. "Many of these words have been too long out of use; if we don't take care of them, they will die." Serving as an advocate for the people in rural communities is one of the writer's premises. She also includes the family in her own narrative: "I am here because of all those women in my family who had no choice, who have been working and who are not visible because they have not had a paid job when they must do all the housework. I want these women to feel recognized, so for me, the book is a kind of loudspeaker," she said, "bringing attention to all aspects of the rural community." In addition to writing, Sánchez continues to work as a veterinarian, since animals are part of her life and she considers them her teachers as well.

As I translated this book I found myself surprised by the linguistic nuances particular to Sánchez's prose, and after investigating them I realized that I too once used language in a similarly nuanced way. Her voice does not have the polish of typical literary nonfiction one often encounters with mainstream Spanish writing; instead, hers is an idiom that is clear and precise, though seemingly awkward at times because of structures that appear and syntactic constructions that are unique to the rural community. Her prose is a result of a language experience connected to the land and the people who work there, a language experience I too had forgotten I once possessed. I am also drawn to her ability to make connections between the natural world and the literary, to compare the overlooked rural stories and the silenced narratives of women in rural communities, and I admire her ability to blend her personal narrative with a movement to give greater attention to rural communities and their inhabitants, in particular women. She writes about her grandmother, for example, whose only schooling was four days in a school for illiterates, and how her grandmother knows how to prepare a garden, save seeds from one year to the next, heal trees, care for animals, make bread. She knows how to do many things that we have lost the ability to do today in our societies, such as understand basic elements of food sovereignty, self-care, and self-management—knowledge she did not acquire at any university but learned from living her life connected to the natural world.

Sánchez does not idealize rural life or the lives of these women so important in her development, but she offers up their stories—stories concerned with ecology, what we consume, climate change, and the social and political crisis we live in—as models for us to rethink our idea of community and common spaces, to see education and culture differently, and to understand that we can learn from each other if we simply take the time to ask questions and listen, especially to "those who have a voice and think that theirs is not worth listening to."